S0-BAX-826

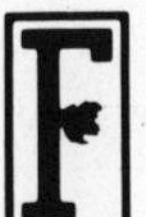

New Ways to Lower Your Blood Pressure

Easy, Safe, Fast Methods That Work

Claire Safran

A Fireside Book
Published by Simon & Schuster, Inc.
New York

A Fireside Book
Published by Simon & Schuster, Inc.
Simon & Schuster Building
Rockefeller Center
1230 Avenue of the Americas
New York, New York 10020
FIRESIDE and colophon are registered trademarks of
Simon & Schuster, Inc.
Designed by Levavi & Levavi
Manufactured in the United States of America

18 17 16 15 14 13 12

Library of Congress Cataloging in Publication Data
Safran, Claire.
New ways to lower your blood pressure.

"A Fireside book,"
1. Hypertension—Prevention. 2. Medicine,
Popular. I. Title.
RC685.H8S24 1984 616.1'32 84-5604
ISBN: 0-671-50380-4

Contents

Foreword

by Thomas G. Pickering, M.D.
Hypertension Center
New York Hospital–Cornell University
Medical Center

New Ways to Lower Your Blood Pressure is a very timely book. In recent years, the public has become increasingly aware of the problems caused by high blood pressure, and this awareness has been heightened by evidence that treating people with high blood pressure, whether mild or severe, can prolong life.

High blood pressure, also known as hypertension, is not a disease in the ordinary sense of the word but a *risk factor.* In this way, it differs from other diseases, such as pneumonia, which you either have or you don't have.

What is meant by a risk factor? It is not itself a disease, but it increases the probability of developing disease. High blood pressure, high blood cholesterol, and smoking are the main risk factors in coronary heart disease, the most frequent cause of death in this country, which is caused by the deposition of plaques that block the coronary arteries supplying the heart muscle.

The reason doctors are concerned about high blood pressure is that, if left unchecked, it increases the probability of heart attack or stroke. If treated with medication, the risk of stroke is reduced, as shown by overwhelming evidence, but we are less certain about protection against heart attack.

There is no exact dividing line between normal and high blood pressure. Your blood pressure is continually changing from moment to moment, and it varies according to what you are doing, thinking, eating, and also according to various chemical and physiological processes occurring inside your body. As to the cause of high blood pressure, there is no simple answer, nor is there likely to be one.

Several factors contribute to the development of high blood pressure, and different mechanisms predominate in different people. In 10 percent of the cases, there is a clearly definable cause, such as a disorder of an adrenal gland or a narrowing of the artery to one of the kidneys. These people are lucky because their blood pressure can be cured permanently either by surgery or renal angioplasty, a procedure whereby the narrowing of the blood vessel can be widened by passing a catheter with an inflatable balloon on its tip across the constriction, and then inflating the balloon. The majority of patients, however, have essential hypertension, for which the underlying cause is unknown, and treatment usually involves the taking of medication indefinitely. Here, different mechanisms can be identified by a test: renin-sodium profiling. This helps determine the type of treatment that is likely to be most effective in a particular case.

There is considerable disagreement among physicians about the best treatment for high blood pressure. First, is any treatment necessary? Since high blood pressure usually causes no symptoms, the decision must be based on the risk level imposed by the raised blood pressure. If the pressure is very high, the increased risk is great, and there is no dispute that drug treatment is indicated. If it is only slightly raised, however, the additional risk is small. In such cases, which constitute the majority of people who have high blood pressure, the practice is to measure the pressure on repeated occasions to ensure a sustained elevation of pressure.

For the same reason, it is important to obtain measurements taken away from the clinic setting, for example, at home and at work. There are many people whose pressure goes up when they visit a doctor but is normal at other times, and most of these people do not need treatment.

Other than the level of pressure, another consideration in recommending treatment is the presence or absence of other cardiovascular risk factors. The harmful effects of high blood pressure are much greater if you also have high blood cholesterol, high blood sugar, or are a heavy smoker. If you don't have any other risk factors, you are less likely to receive treatment for mild high blood pressure.

The next step is deciding the treatment that is most appropriate for you. With a good history and physical examination, and a few simple tests such as a renin-sodium profile, the physician can identify the small percentage (5–10 percent) who have curable hypertension. For the rest, the physician will choose either a pharmacological (drug) or non-pharmacological treatment. The latter is preferable because it avoids the cost and side effects of drug treatment. Because hypertension stems from different causes in different patients, one form of treatment may work very well for one, but not for another. For example, if you are going to try a sodium-restricted diet, try it for a few weeks and then have your pressure rechecked. If it is not lower at the end of this period, either you haven't lowered your intake of sodium enough (this is easily checked by measuring the urine sodium) or you are not "sodium sensitive," and there is little point in continuing the diet.

New Ways to Lower Your Blood Pressure appropriately emphasizes methods that you can do for yourself, other than just taking medication, such as diet, exercise, and relaxation techniques. Remember that everyone is different: not all treatments will be equally successful in your case. One of the best ways of checking your progress is to learn how to measure your own blood pressure at home. These records will be helpful to you and your doctor. You will get the best results if both of you work as a team. As Claire Safran points out, one of the most important steps toward lowering your blood pressure is to take control and educate yourself about high blood pressure.

1. You and Your Doctor

"You're writing a book about blood pressure?" my neighbor asks. "A whole book?"

He has high blood pressure, and the information his doctor has handed him fills one side of a single sheet of paper. That's all the doctor thought he needed to know. That's all the doctor—with a waiting room filled with other impatient patients—had time to offer him.

Yet there's more—much more—that anyone with high blood pressure needs to know. The more you know and understand, the better and the sooner you will be able to lower your blood pressure.

If you have high blood pressure, you need to be under a doctor's care. This book is not a substitute for a visit to your doctor. It is a stand-in for the questions your doctor may not have had time to answer. Or the questions you forgot to ask. Or the ones you didn't know enough to ask.

The best patient is an educated patient. You are the one who will pay the price for a blood pressure that's too high. You're also the one who will reap the rewards of a blood pressure that's healthy.

You and your doctor ought to be partners in deciding

about your care and treatment. To be an active partner, you need to know what the problems are, and what choices you have in dealing with those problems. To get the best answers from your doctor, you need to know what questions to ask.

This book, then, is for my neighbor. Armed with a single piece of paper and a prescription for some pills, he isn't controlling his high blood pressure—or hypertension, as it's also called. There are no symptoms with hypertension. Because he doesn't feel sick, he forgets to take his pills. Because he doesn't understand why he should make some changes in his life-style, he also forgets about the other things on his piece of paper. Indeed, if you ask him, he'll tell you, with a sheepish grin, that he's lost the piece of paper.

This book is also for my mother, a kind and gentle woman who became a martyr to her blood pressure. For decades, a cluster of pill bottles was the centerpiece of her breakfast table. Religiously, she took her medicine and swallowed her bland diet. She worried about her pressure, brooded about it, sacrificed too many of life's pleasures on its altar. She cut out salt but she added anxiety, which was just as bad for her blood pressure.

It is also for my husband, who tried to take the opposite path when the doctor told him his blood pressure was too high. He winked away the problem—at his own risk. For a year, he drove his doctor—and his wife—crazy. Then he found a way to feel good, live well—and still lower his pressure. He did it without drugs and without a life-souring diet.

There are forty to sixty million Americans like my mother, like my husband, like my neighbor. Their blood pressure is too high, putting their lives in danger. High blood pressure, or hypertension, isn't really a disease. It's more of a symptom, like fever. It's a sign that something is wrong.

High blood pressure has been called the silent killer. Few people die of the high blood pressure itself, but a great many do pass away because of its fatal consequences. If left ignored and untreated, high blood pressure can become a major cause of the leading killers of our time—heart attacks, strokes, and kidney failure.

Yet that doesn't need to happen. Today, anyone with high

blood pressure can bring it down. Doctors have not just one way to help you do that but several. And you can do it quickly. It may have taken years for your blood pressure to climb to where it is now. Yet it can begin to come down in just thirty days—and probably sooner.

The tragedy is not that so many people have high blood pressure. It's that so few are doing anything about it. Some don't know they have it. Others know they have it but don't know enough about the treatment that would be best for them.

Only about one out of every three people who have hypertension is controlling it, according to Dr. Edward Rocella of the National Heart, Lung, and Blood Institute, one of the National Institutes of Health. That's a small percentage, but a decade ago it was only one in five. The change is enough to have an effect that can be measured. The number of deaths caused by strokes has fallen dramatically. The number of fatal heart attacks is edging down. Lives are being saved because people are paying attention to their systolic (the upper number in your blood-pressure reading) and their diastolic (the lower number).

This book is also for myself. My blood pressure is 120 over 80, a good, healthy, "normal" reading. Yet, I, too, am at risk. My pressure could climb higher, especially since one of my parents had high blood pressure. I'm a candidate for edging up to a diastolic in the 90's or higher, but that, too, doesn't need to happen. People like me can practice preventive medicine. Some of the methods for lowering blood pressure are not only lifesaving, they're life-enhancing. Without waiting until we get sick, people like me can use those methods now.

Once upon a time, there was only one thing that doctors could do about high blood pressure. They would prescribe a bland diet of boiled rice, relieved only by some fruit. No wonder so few people stayed with the "cure."

Today, the picture is very different. There's now a range of remedies and methods for lowering the blood pressure. For each person, a treatment can be tailored to fit who you are, how you live, and how high your pressure is.

Some people may wonder why a medical book isn't being written by a medical person. The answer is a question: Which medical person? Which doctor?

There has been an explosion of research on high blood pressure in recent years. Different doctors, though, embrace different bits and pieces of the research. Different doctors would write very different books.

The debate about the results of the recent research is heated. It is enough to raise anyone's blood pressure. It swirls around the basic issues of health care, no matter what the disease. Do we experiment with new ideas or stick with the tried-and-tested ones? How much is in your mind, and how much in your body? What part do you play in your own cure, and what do you leave to the doctor?

Some researchers blame high blood pressure on your parents and on the genes they gave you. Others say you can "catch it" from your husband, your boss, your life-style. Some say that salt is the villain in this disease; others insist that salt is innocent and may even be good for you. Some claim that today's pills work like a charm; others say that the most powerful medicine is in your head.

Who's right? For an individual patient, the answers have to be worked out with a doctor you can trust. It helps if it's a doctor who will take the time to know you, because your spirit as well as your body counts in any illness. It helps, too, if you will take the time to know what questions to ask, because that's always the path to the best answers about your health.

In this book, we'll be sorting out the research and looking at the new information, new ideas, new approaches, and new treatments.

We'll be following what the wisest doctors say—that you don't treat the disease, you treat the patient.

We'll be telling you about a range of remedies and a repertoire of cures—so that you can talk to your doctor about the one that's right for you.

Let's see now what the questions about blood pressure—and the answers—are. There are a number of roads back to health. Which is the best path for you?

2. What Is High Blood Pressure?

The body rings no alarms and signals no symptoms. There is no pain, no wound that you can see, no sense of being sick.

One day, you are feeling just fine. The next day, in a routine examination, the doctor wraps a black cuff around your arm and pumps it up. Seconds later, the doctor is frowning at a column of mercury that has stayed too high in the measuring device, the sphygmomanometer. And then you are given the bad news.

You have high blood pressure.
Or someone you love has it.
And what then?

What the Numbers Mean

The doctor measures your blood pressure by stopping the pressure—and then starting it again. The cuff is wrapped around your upper arm and inflated, cutting off the flow of blood in the main artery. Then, as the doctor deflates the cuff, letting out the air, the blood begins to flow again.

The force of the blood at that moment is the systolic pressure, the upper number in your blood-pressure reading. The artery is filled with blood and is at its highest pressure. Then, as the blood continues to flow, the artery relaxes. The force of the blood at that moment is the diastolic pressure, the lower number in your blood-pressure reading.

Both numbers, systolic and diastolic, upper and lower, are important. If either is too high, you have hypertension. For the average adult, a healthy blood pressure reading is 120 over 80—or lower. For someone with high blood pressure, the reading might be 160 over 95—or higher.

In most people, the numbers depend one on the other. They are intimately connected, going up and down together, working in tandem. That's why so many people—both physicians and patients—often find it simpler to talk about just one number, the lower or diastolic reading.

Here is what your diastolic is saying:

If it is 115 or above, you have severe hypertension. This is the red zone, highly dangerous.

If it is between 105 and 114, you're in the yellow zone that doctors call moderate hypertension.

If it's 95 to 104, you have mild hypertension. This is the gray area, the place where doctors disagree among themselves over what the best treatment is.

If it's 90 to 94, you have borderline hypertension. Together with those in the mild range, this is where three-fourths of the people with high blood pressure find themselves.

If it's 80 to 89, you're in what used to be considered a normal and safe range. Today, though, there are new warning flags about a diastolic in the 80's. More and more doctors think it ought to be checked regularly, to be sure it doesn't edge into the 90's.

Later in this chapter, we'll be talking about the risk factors for higher blood pressure. If you have one or more of these, it can make mild or borderline high blood pressure more serious than it seems. A diastolic reading in the 80's could be a signal to start doing something about it, preventing the disease now rather than waiting until you have to cure it later.

Can It Ever Be Too Low?

When it comes to blood pressure, the lower, the healthier. "It can never be too low," says Dr. Thomas G. Pickering of the Hypertension Center at The New York Hospital–Cornell Medical Center in New York City. As he notes, the only exception is if you feel dizzy or faint when you change positions from lying down to sitting up, or from sitting down to standing up.

If that happens, you should consult your doctor. Some people with low blood pressure complain of feeling tired all the time, and that's another thing to talk to your doctor about. The cause may be something other than blood pressure.

Mostly, if you have low blood pressure, a diastolic in the 60's or 70's, doctors think you should count yourself lucky—and plan on surviving to a ripe and wonderful age. How does living to be a hundred and twenty sound?

That Other Number

The numbers that define the different ranges of blood pressure are lower today than they once were. Now that there are so many different ways to bring the pressure down—in many cases *without* drugs—doctors are beginning to worry about it earlier. The sooner we do something, the better—and the easier—they now believe.

Most of the research on blood pressure shows that they're right to believe that. Most of the research also focuses on the diastolic, or lower number, and in this book we'll be talking mostly about the diastolic.

Yet the other number, the systolic, shouldn't be forgotten completely. It's at least as important as the diastolic. Usually, they zig and zag together, but there are cases where the systolic takes off by itself.

It used to be thought that the systolic *had* to go up with age, but that's been disproved. It used to be believed that a healthy systolic was 100 plus the person's age. Now we know that a systolic of 165 is probably too high for a person of 65 years. Ideally, both numbers should stay down, no matter what the birthday.

Sometimes, the lower number will be just fine but the systolic will be way up there. That's called "systolic hypertension," and it happens mostly in elderly people. It's a medical puzzle, but a too high systolic often seems to respond to the same kinds of treatments that doctors use for a too high diastolic.

Who Gets High Blood Pressure?

When as many as sixty million Americans may have the same disease, it's fair to say that anyone can get it. It is a democratic, nondiscriminating problem. Within that truth, though, there are patterns that are worth looking at.

The Sex Difference: One of the myths about high blood pressure is that women get it more than men do. The reality is the opposite—but not exactly. Until about age forty-five, fewer women than men have high blood pressure. When those younger women do have it, they have it less severely than men do. Women also tolerate it better. Until their mid-forties, many women seem to have a built-in protection against the dangerous outcomes of high blood pressure, especially against heart attacks.

Young women who are taking the birth-control pill, which can raise the blood pressure slightly, should be especially careful to have their pressure checked regularly. Other women may get high blood pressure when they are pregnant. It's vital to treat this, for the health of both mother and baby. After the birth, though, this kind of high blood pressure usually goes away.

In their mid-forties, women seem to lose their earlier protection. Now they begin to catch up with men and eventually pass them on high blood pressure. Among the elderly, more women than men have it.

Doctors aren't certain why the sex difference exists. The special protection that women have and then lose could be connected to their hormonal makeup and the changes that take place in it during menopause. Or it could be life-style. Today, more and more women are living more like men, doing both constructive things like striving for a career and destructive ones like smoking. Some doctors think women may begin to get high blood pressure and heart attacks just as men do, too.

The Age Factor: High blood pressure is thought of as an old-age disease, but that's half myth, half truth. Because they've lived longer, older people have had more time for their blood pressure to climb to higher levels. Thus their pressure may be higher than that of younger people.

The problem, though, begins earlier, in the middle years. For most people, high blood pressure starts between age thirty and age fifty. If you don't get it during those years, you may never get it. Yet you may have it during those years and not know it. Since there are no warnings or symptoms, many people don't discover they have high blood pressure until they're much older—and the pressure is that much higher. That's why it's important to have your blood pressure checked regularly—at any age.

Once, it was believed that blood pressure *had* to go up with age, that old people needed that extra pressure to keep functioning. Indeed, it used to be called *essential hypertension.* Today we know that it's neither essential nor healthy, and that pressure can be lowered and kept lowered at any age.

When Children Get It: Generally, high blood pressure is an adult rather than a childhood disease. Still, it has been found even in very young babies and it can happen in children. Today, good pediatricians check blood pressure as part of a child's routine examination.

Some children develop secondary high blood pressure, the kind that's caused by other diseases such as heart or kidney disease. If the other disease is treated successfully, the child's pressure usually goes back down to normal.

Other children develop primary high blood pressure, the kind that is not linked to other diseases, the form that most adults have. These children may have some of the risk factors that we'll be talking about next. If a child's blood pressure goes up only a small amount, it may be something the child will "outgrow."If the child consistently has blood pressure that is higher than the average and also has one or more risk factors, it may be that that child will also have high blood pressure as an adult. Child or adult, there are many ways to bring the pressure down and continue to live a full and normal life.

An Unequal-Opportunity Disease: Black Americans, more than any other group, develop high blood pressure. Though one out of six Americans has it, it's one out of four for blacks. Some researchers would put that as high as one out of three blacks.

For blacks, it could be something genetic. High blood pressure does run in families and could be hereditary. Some researchers report that there's a difference in high blood pressure among blacks whose ancestors come from different parts of Africa.

It could also be something in the environment. Stress is a factor in high blood pressure, and in our society blacks are under more stress than other people. As a group, they live with more crowding, more poverty, more tension, more sense of being the stranger, the outsider, than do other groups of people.

Your Risk Profile

There are a number of factors that make it more likely that you will develop high blood pressure. There are other factors that can make the disease more dangerous to your health.

Test your own risk quotient with these questions:

Does It Run in Your Family? Do one or both of your parents have high blood pressure? A brother or sister? There's a hereditary factor to high blood pressure. Still, as Dr. Pickering says, it's a "graded" inheritance. That means that if your parents have it, you'll probably have it, too, but your pressure won't necessarily be as high as theirs.

What is it that you inherit? It's not clear yet whether a genetic fault, a weakness in the blood vessels, is passed on from generation to generation. It's obvious that we inherit more than genes and chromosomes from our parents. Home is where we learn about eating—and perhaps overeating. It's where we pick up preferences for some foods over others. It's where our emotions are shaped, our ways of reacting to the world around us, our patterns of dealing with stress. The family environment is a large part of our inheritance.

Indeed, recent research by Dr. Sydney Stahl of Purdue University suggests that you can "catch" high blood pressure from your husband or wife. He's found that some married couples get it together. Or one develops high blood pressure and the other has migraines. "They share the same stresses," he explains. "So if one of them is talking through his body, the other will find a way to talk, too."

Are you overweight? Too many pounds can lead to too much blood pressure. Being overweight can be a strain on your circulatory system, and so cause the blood pressure to rise. It also makes having high blood pressure a more serious, more dangerous condition, since you're now dealing with a combination of two major threats for heart attacks.

Do you have diabetes? Diabetes doesn't cause hypertension, but it often goes along with being overweight, which does cause it. Diabetes also has been implicated in heart disease, so diabetes and high blood pressure each add to the danger of the other.

Do you have high cholesterol? High levels of cholesterol can make the blood pressure go high, too. The cholesterol can clog the blood vessels with a fatty residue, narrowing the passage, raising the force that's needed to move the blood along. If you have both high cholesterol and high blood pressure, you are especially vulnerable to the possibility of heart attack or stroke. There's some evidence that a tendency to high cholesterol is hereditary. So even if you don't have it but have a parent who does, now's the time to do something about your diet—and your blood pressure.

Do you smoke? Cigarettes don't cause high blood pressure, but they are a synergism. When you add smoking to hypertension, you're not just adding one major danger of heart attack to another, you're multiplying the dangers. If you stop smoking, it may not lower your blood pressure, but it will lower the danger and it will improve your health in many other ways. Until you do manage to kick the habit, it's vital to do something about your blood pressure.

Are you a type-A person? Are you a driving, striving person? Highly ambitious? A workaholic? A perfectionist? These traits are typical of what scientists call the type-A personality. Such people don't get higher blood pressure than other people, but it's riskier for them. The type-A personality is implicated in heart disease, and researchers are finding that people with high blood pressure who also are type-A's are more susceptible to heart attacks. It's another red-flag warning to bring your pressure down.

Are you under stress? It doesn't matter where you live, what kind of work you do, how you spend your days and nights. If you feel you are under stress, then that's what you are—under stress and at risk. The link between stress and high blood pressure is becoming clearer and clearer, and it's important to bring the levels of both down.

How to Use This Book

Knowledge is one of the world's best medicines. It can help you to understand what's happening in your body, and it can point out the roads to changing and improving it. It can give you a precious gift—a sense of being in control of your own health and destiny, a mental attitude that leads to physical health.

That's why I hope that everyone will read all of this book. The more you know about your blood pressure, the better you can control it. Still, the book doesn't need to be read in the order of its numbered pages. It's designed so that you can skip ahead to a section that applies especially to you, as you are today. Then you can turn back to other sections, to complete your personal story.

Different sections of this book will help different people get started faster on lowering their blood pressure. Remember, though, any change you plan to make—especially in diet, exercise, or medication—should be discussed with your doctor first.

Find the description or descriptions that fit you; then turn first to the suggested chapter or chapters.

If your pressure is 105 or higher, turn first to Chapter 4, which discusses drugs that can save your life. Then read the chapters on diet, on lowering salt, on exercise, and on relaxation—to make those drugs work even better.

If it's 95 to 104, read Chapter 4 on drugs. Then learn about some of the new nondrug therapies, such as those in Chapters 5, 10, 11, and 14.

If it's 90 to 94, turn to Chapters 5, 6, and 7 for ideas on how to change your blood pressure by changing what you eat. Read Chapters 11 through 14, which tell how to use your head to lower your pressure. Don't miss Chapter 10, to learn how to run away from hypertension.

If it's 80 to 89, Chapters 10 through 14 will tell you how to keep it that healthy way with new, effective preventive therapies.

If your doctor has advised you to lose weight, turn to Chapter 5 for a diet that isn't really a diet and to Chapter 6 for ideas on "cooking smart."

If you feel you're under stress, Chapters 11 through 14 can provide new and effective ways to deal with it. Chapter 10 can also help you.

If you're a type-A person, read Chapter 14 on managing your anger.

If your doctor has prescribed a lower-salt diet, Chapter 7 will tell you how to shake the salt habit—without tears. Chapters 5 and 6 also have good ideas for you.

If your doctor has advised you to eat more potassium, see Chapter 9.

If you wonder what kind of high blood pressure you have, see Chapters 8 and 9.

3. What the Doctor Didn't Tell You

A visit to the doctor's office is enough to raise anyone's blood pressure. You feel nervous, worried about what's wrong with you, and that pushes up your pressure.

Or you are one of those people who see the doctor as authority-in-a-white-coat, and talking to an authority figure—like a doctor, like a boss—will raise your pressure.

Or perhaps you're worried about how you're going to pay the bill, and that's what's causing your pressure to go up.

Doctors understand these things. Most good doctors will want to take your blood pressure on more than one visit, to get a truer picture of it before prescribing.

Meanwhile, though, are you getting the information that you need? Among themselves, doctors complain about what they call the compliance problem—the great numbers of patients who don't follow the doctor's orders. Recent research shows that patients who understand the problem are more likely to follow the prescription. Knowledge is the great motivator.

What, then, is going on, if you have high blood pressure? What is it that's happening in your body? What's really wrong with you?

The Life Force

Blood pressure is vital to life. It's a way of measuring the force that it takes to keep the blood moving along on its journey through your body, a trip that goes, literally, from head to toe. Each of us has about five quarts of blood, and that entire supply circulates through the body about once a minute. That's the equivalent of moving nine or ten tons of blood every twenty-four hours.

The heart of this system is the human heart. That's the pump that starts and controls the movement of blood. About seventy times a minute, a healthy heart pumps or beats. With each beat, the heart pushes out half a cup of blood, starting it on its way through the arteries (the major blood vessels), the arterioles (the smaller, more elastic blood vessels), and the capillaries (the thinnest vessels of all, the ones that deliver the blood's cargo of oxygen and nutrients to the body's cells).

It's a lightning-quick journey—but a long one, through more than sixty thousand miles of blood vessels. At each step, the blood vessel expands, filling up with blood. Then it contracts, to send the blood along. The pressure in the blood vessel when it's expanded is the systolic or upper number of your blood-pressure reading. The pressure when it's contracted or relaxed is the diastolic or lower number.

How the Numbers Change

Dozens and dozens of times a day, your blood pressure changes. Depending on what you're doing and how you're feeling, it goes up or down.

The circulatory system is a sensitive one, and it reacts quickly to help you carry on your activities. If you're running, it detours an extra bonus of blood to your legs, to speed you on your way. If you're eating, the extra blood is rerouted to the stomach, to aid with digestion.

If you're moving about, your blood pressure is higher than when you're sitting still. It goes up when you're angry and subsides when you're happy. For almost everyone, it's higher during the eight hours that you are at work than during the time when you're at home.

Researchers at The New York Hospital–Cornell Medical Center wired a group of patients with portable electronic blood-pressure recorders. When they matched those records with the diaries that people kept of what they were doing, they had a twenty-four-hour picture of how blood pressure rises and falls. Here's how, on the average, different activities affect and change the systolic pressure (the first number) and the diastolic pressure (the second number):

Sex—plus 31/11
Drinking—plus 12/5
Eating—plus 3/3
Shopping—plus 6/2
Telephoning—plus 2/2
Sleeping—minus 17/12
Reading—minus 7/4
Relaxing—minus 13/9
Watching TV—minus 8/6
Listening to music—minus 5/4

Your blood pressure changes with what you're feeling as well as with what you're doing. It zigs and zags with big stresses and little ones, real dangers and imagined ones. Do you need to swerve your car suddenly, to avoid hitting a child who's run out into the road? Are you telephoning someone of the opposite sex to ask for a date? Are you worried about whether your guests will enjoy themselves at your party? Are you upset because someone is keeping you waiting? Or are you rushing because you're the one who's late?

Daily life is filled with routine ups and downs, and your blood pressure rises and falls along with them. That's natural and normal. For people with high blood pressure, though, the swings are wider, the highs are higher, and the lows aren't low enough. The strain on the system is greater, more frequent, and more constant. Until you learn to control it, that's the danger of high blood pressure.

If Something Goes Wrong . . .

Whatever the byways and detours, the peaks and valleys, the journey always ends where it started, at the heart. Here the blood is drawn in once again, cleansed and refreshed with oxygen, and then sent out on another round trip.

A blood-pressure reading is a way of describing how that trip is going. If the path is smooth and clear, if extra pressure isn't needed to expand and contract the blood vessels, then the reading will be a healthy and normal one. If the path is difficult, if it is narrowed or partly blocked in places, then the blood vessels—and also the heart—have to work harder. The blood-pressure reading will be higher. The extra points are the extra pressure that it took for the vessels to move the blood along.

The body is a marvelous machine. Within it, the amount of work performed by the circulatory system is prodigious. Writing about blood pressure, Dr. Max L. Feinman looks at the work the heart does over an average lifetime. He estimates that if that effort were concentrated in a single moment, it could lift about four hundred and fifty million pounds—the equivalent weight of the entire population of Chicago and its surrounding suburbs.

Still, like any machine, this one will last longer if it is not overworked. Your car may be capable of going one hundred miles per hour, but you know it will serve you longer if your usual speed is a more moderate one. It's the same with your bodily machine. High blood pressure pushes it to the limits—or beyond—straining the system, making it falter, sputter, fail.

If blood pressure stays too high for too long, the artery walls can become weakened. Eventually, there may be a blowout, and this seems to happen most often in the most vital area—the brain. Or the artery may become clogged, unable to feed the cells that depend on it. Those cells will then starve to death. Again, this usually happens in the brain. Whichever way it happens, these are two forms of a terrible event—a stroke.

Sometimes, it is like a hydraulic system gone awry. The

pump—in this case, your heart—rebels. If the heart muscle has to work against an ever greater resistance or pressure in the arteries, the muscle responds by thickening. Eventually, the heart weakens, enlarges, dilates, and that can lead to heart failure.

These two prognoses are bleak, indeed. Yet neither needs to come true for you. It is never too early or too late to lower your blood pressure.

How It Begins

Doctors aren't sure why blood pressure creeps up and up in some people but not in others. They're not certain when it begins to happen. Yet happen it does.

Being overweight can do it for some people. The more you weigh, the more cells there are for your circulatory system to feed. That means it has to work harder, under greater pressure.

Whatever you weigh, a high-fat diet can lead to high blood pressure. This is the core of the cholesterol problem. If there are high levels of fat in the blood, then, as it moves through the blood vessels, it leaves behind a thin, waxy streak, a deposit of cholesterol and other fats. With time, that streak builds up along the inner wall of the blood vessel. The path gets narrower and narrower, and the blood pressure gets higher and higher. This can happen to any artery but it seems to happen most often to the arteries that lead in and out of the heart. So, along with high blood pressure, you may have coronary atherosclerosis. That means the heart's arteries are thickened with fatty deposits, narrowed, and under great strain—a condition that can lead to a heart attack.

If the heart is the pump of the body's hydraulic system, the kidney is a monitor. One of its jobs is to guard the blood pressure, triggering extra hormones to raise the pressure when it drops too low. If the kidney is blocked or damaged by disease, though, it may send out a call for those hormones even when they're not needed by the rest of the body—thus causing high blood pressure.

It's the kidney's job, too, to deal with the salt in your system and to excrete the excess salt and water. In some people, though, the kidneys get their hormonal messages crossed, and they don't process the salt as they should. These people may not consume more salt than other people do, but their salt just stays there. Then the sodium, a major ingredient in common salt, grabs water. This causes the blood volume and the tissue volume to expand. In turn, that forces the body to use more pressure to keep the blood circulating.

In other people, according to new research, the problem starts with renin, a substance produced by the kidneys. Renin plays a role in regulating the blood pressure, not directly but indirectly, by starting a series of hormonal effects. Among the substances it summons is a powerful one called angiotensin II, a hormone that tells the kidney to hold on to sodium. That starts the process of holding on to water, expanding the blood and tissue volume . . . and raising the pressure.

Today, medical science is beginning to follow other clues and track down other causes. There is a new research frontier—it concerns substances in your body called ions, such minerals as calcium, potassium, and magnesium. Too little of some of these ions, or too much of others, can be a factor in raising the blood pressure.

For a few people, the cause is physical. A blockage or injury to the kidneys or to the arteries leading to and from them can interfere with the circulation of the blood and send the pressure soaring. Surgery may be called for in these cases, and there now are new procedures that are simpler and safer than ever.

In Your Mind

Hypertension is not the same as tension, but they often go hand in glove. In different people, mental stress may make itself felt in the body in different ways. Some people develop ulcers. Other people may get migraine headaches. And many people get high blood pressure.

Blood pressure is a key part of the body's remarkable, all-purpose system for dealing with stresses, challenges, emergencies. If you're running, for example, your heart speeds up, your breathing comes faster, your blood pressure rises—all to provide the muscles with what they need to run.

That's appropriate. The same revving up takes place, though, when physical activity isn't called for, when the stress is emotional or psychological. Modern life is full of such stresses. The alarm clock goes off. The phone jangles. The dinner burns. You argue with someone. In reaction to such small daily events, your mind sends your body into high gear. The higher your blood pressure is to start with, though, the higher the gear you may go into. And the greater the strain on your system.

The Good News

There are still questions about blood pressure for which doctors have no answers, but they have more answers today than ever before. There are new drugs and new diets. New ways to deal with stress. New ideas about salt. New approaches to ion imbalances. New procedures for surgery. For every suspected cause, there's now a way to correct it and control your blood pressure.

Indeed, for most people, as we'll see, there's more than one way.

4. Drugs That Can Save Your Life

The doctor reaches for a pad and pen and writes out a prescription. You probably can't read the handwriting but it spells "lifesaver." The doctor has ordered one or more of the medications that can lower almost anybody's blood pressure.

Drugs are the surest of all the blood-pressure remedies. They are the quickest. Some can bring blood pressure back to normal *in a matter of days!*

Why, then, doesn't everyone with high blood pressure just take a pill?

Rx: Not for Everyone

As we said, there has been an explosion of research on high blood pressure—and a fallout of medical debate and disagreement. You may have read some of the reports on this research in your newspaper, and found the headlines confusing. Yet it's important to straighten out the major findings.

If you have a diastolic of 105 or higher, there's no argument and no confusion. Just about all the research shows that medication is the most certain and swiftest way to bring your pressure down to safe limits. Just about any doctor will prescribe medication for you, though your doctor may also urge other things to do along with taking the pills.

If you have a diastolic of 90 to 104, you're in the great majority of hypertensives. You're also the patient whom everyone is arguing about. This is the gray area, where different research comes up with different findings.

In recent years, there have been two major reports of long-term population research on high blood pressure. Until their findings were made known, most doctors were prescribing drugs for moderate and severe cases of hypertension. For mild and borderline cases, most weren't writing prescriptions; instead, the usual treatment was to urge these patients to lose weight, cut back on salt or cholesterol, stop smoking, or make some other life-style change.

Then the research results were announced, and doctors began arguing among themselves. The findings were contradictory, but each side had a number of smaller studies to use as confirmation of its views.

The Hypertension and Detection Follow-Up Program (HDFP) was a five-year, $70 million study involving more than ten thousand people with high blood pressure. Like the general population, the great majority of these patients, more than seventy percent of them, were in the mild or borderline zones.

The people in the study were divided into two groups. One group had intensive care; drugs were prescribed for them, and they were given free care at special clinics—and with free transportation, if they needed it. The other group was referred to local doctors, and the milder cases were given the usual nondrug treatment.

HDFP confirmed the value of drugs for moderate and severe cases. Those who were given the intensive and free care were less likely to drop away from the treatment than were those in the second group. They were also less likely to suffer the fatal outcomes of high blood pressure, such as heart attacks and strokes.

The study also seemed to show that drugs were a good idea for the mild and borderline cases. Those under the intensive care, with drugs, did better than those under the usual nondrug care.

Some doctors began to rush to write prescriptions for their milder cases. Other doctors said, "Wait a minute!" Was it the drugs that made the difference for the milder cases? Or was it the difference between intensive and free care versus usual care?

A while after the HDFP, the results were announced for another major study. Mr. Fit, the nickname for the Multiple Risk Factor Intervention Trial, was a ten-year study, costing $115 million, that also involved thousands of people with hypertension. In this study, drugs were a lifesaver for those with higher pressure, but they seemed to have a bad effect on the milder cases. In Mr. Fit, the milder cases who were treated *without* drugs did better than those who got them.

Who Should Get Drugs?

As doctors look again and again at the research, a consensus is emerging:

For a diastolic over 105, almost every doctor will prescribe drugs.

For a diastolic between 100 and 104, some doctors will put the patient on drugs; others will try other nondrug treatments first.

For a diastolic under 100, most doctors will try nondrug treatments first, always keeping a careful eye on the patient and his or her blood pressure.

Dr. Edward Freis of the Veterans Administration is a pioneer in blood-pressure research, especially in the early research that proved how effective drugs can be for people with severe hypertension. Today, along with many other doctors, he worries that the drug cure for milder cases can be riskier than the diseases.

"Unless there are other risk factors," says Dr. Freis, "the danger in mild hypertension is so low that drugs are not warranted."

Good doctors, as we said, treat the patient rather than the disease. So they weigh the risk factors. Is there a family history of severe high blood pressure? Is the patient overweight? A diabetic? A smoker? If one or more risk factors are there, the doctor may prescribe drugs even for a milder case—especially if the patient is unwilling to lower the risk factor by changing his or her habits.

There is new evidence, published in a recent issue of the *Journal of the American Medical Association,* about drugs and the type-A personality. These are the men and women who may be workaholics, perfectionists, self-drivers, compulsive strivers. West German physicians are finding in their research that the behavior of type-A people changes when they are given one class of blood-pressure drugs, beta-blockers. Type-A behavior, as we've said, doesn't cause high blood pressure, but it is a co-risk for heart disease. So some doctors now are giving these drugs even to mild cases, if the type-A risk factor is there.

There's one risk factor, though, that pushes doctors away from drugs rather than toward them. Mr. Fit showed that drugs were especially dangerous for people who had an abnormal EKG (electrocardiogram) along with their mild hypertension. When the two dangers are both there, doctors are particularly careful about what they prescribe.

What Are the Drugs?

For those who need it, the drug treatment is there, and it is remarkably effective. It works for almost anyone who will follow it. And it works faster than anything else. Using the nondrug treatments that we'll be talking about in this book, most people can lower their blood pressure in thirty days. Using the drug treatment, many people can bring their pressure down to normal in just a few days.

The standard treatment is called Stepped Care. It gets that name because it begins with the lowest step, the mildest possible drug and the lowest possible dosage, and works up from there.

Step One is usually a diuretic. This medicine lowers the body's volume of fluid by flushing sodium, which raises that volume, out of the body. That decreases the pressure, and for many people that's all that's needed.

Doctors usually will prescribe a diuretic by such brand names as Diuril, Enduron, Hygroton, Naturetin, Aldactone, Hydromox, Lasix, and a dozen others.

If Step One doesn't bring the pressure down to a safe level, the doctor will add *Step Two.* Traditionally, this has been a beta-blocker, something to calm down the sympathetic nervous system and so ease the pressure.

Among the brand-name drugs that do this are Inderal, Corgard, Lopressor, and a number of others. Serpasil, Ismelin, and Minipress are not beta-blockers, but they also act on the sympathetic nervous system.

For those few patients whose pressure is still too high, *Step Three* is usually a vasodilator. This type of drug relaxes the muscles of the blood-vessel walls, and so lowers the pressure.

Among the brand-name vasodilators that a doctor may prescribe are Loniten, Apresoline, and others. If the pressure still isn't controlled with these medications, even more powerful drugs are available.

New Drugs, New Cures

As science learns more and more about the different forms of high blood pressure, and the different causes, new families of drugs are being developed.

For some people, for example, it is not too much salt that causes the pressure to go up; it's too much renin. Produced by the kidneys, renin affects the blood pressure by setting off a series of hormonal reactions. One of the substances it summons up is a powerful one called angiotensin II. A new drug called captopril can inhibit this effect.

This drug was first available under the brand name of Capoten, but other pharmaceutical companies are now preparing their own versions of this drug. Dr. John Laragh, founder of the Hypertension Center at The New York Hospital, reports that he has been able to totally or partially correct high blood pressure in a very high percentage of cases with this antirenin drug.

For other people, the problem is the way the body handles calcium. Sometimes, too much calcium can accumulate in the blood-vessel walls, causing them to contract so that the blood pressure goes up. A new class of drugs, calcium channel blockers, act as gatekeepers, blocking the calcium from entering into the cells. As we go to press, the Food and Drug Administration has not approved these drugs for blood-pressure treatment yet, but some doctors have begun to prescribe them nevertheless.

What about Side Effects?

Every drug, alas, has its side effects. That's why doctors are careful to prescribe them only for those who need them.

Diuretics, for example, can cause fatigue, muscle weakness, leg cramps, a low potassium level, or an elevated uric acid level. Beta-blockers may slow the heart rate or pulse, aggravate asthma, cause leg cramps, or bring on fatigue or depression. Vasodilators may step up the heart rate and cause headaches, stuffy noses, and fluid retention.

Lists of possible side effects for any drug can be frightening, but the cure is not worse than the disease. Many people don't experience any side effects at all.

For those who do, it's important to discuss them with your doctor. People don't feel sick with high blood pressure. If they then take a medicine that makes them feel worse, some may be tempted to skip taking those pills. Yet that's inviting danger. The wise course is to talk to your doctor. Often, the doctor can adjust the dose or switch from one brand to another, and so eliminate the uncomfortable side effect.

Some medications, for example, can affect your sexual desire or your sexual performance. Doctors tend not to mention this possible side effect. Some are embarrassed to talk about it. Others don't want to influence you; they worry that if they mention the possibility, it's more likely to happen. Yet if it does happen, it's important to talk to the doctor about it, so that the drug or the size of the dose can be switched. Nearly all drug-related effects on sexuality are reversible.

If you're taking blood-pressure drugs, a reassuring word comes from Dr. Edward Freis, who has spent decades caring for patients on these drugs. He says of the side effects, "I haven't seen anything yet to alarm me."

What to Ask Your Doctor

Various surveys have shown that patients take their medications improperly as often as 50 percent of the time. According to a Chilton Research study in 1982 and a Louis Harris survey in 1983, nearly 70 percent of patients were not told about precautions and possible side effects by their doctors. Only 2 to 4 percent of the patients said they had asked questions about their prescriptions while in the doctor's office.

If you're informed about the drug you're taking, you're more likely to stick with it. If you ask questions, you're more apt to get the full benefit of it. Here, then, are questions you should ask about any prescription:

- What is the name of the drug?
- What is it supposed to do?
- What foods, drinks, other medications, and activities should I avoid while taking the drug?
- Should I take the drug before, during, or after meals?
- Are there any side effects, and what should I do if they occur?
- Is there any written information I can take with me?

The "Easy" Pill

The unopened pill bottle doesn't do anyone any good. Yet sometimes because of a side effect, sometimes because they just forget, many people stop taking their medicine or don't take it as often as they should.

Doctors understand that the simpler the regime or medicine, the easier it is to follow. Especially for older people, who may be taking other pills for other problems, the routine can be complicated and confusing.

Now science is beginning to come up with answers for that. Inderal has just become available in a new time-release formula, so that it only needs to be taken once a day. Clonidine is available as an easy-to-use bandage patch. Other pharmaceutical companies will no doubt soon be coming out with easy-to-use formulations of their own beta-blockers and their own versions of the other classes of blood-pressure drugs.

The more you become an active partner in your own health care, the better you'll remember to take your pills. Just about anyone, for example, can learn to take his or her own blood pressure. There are simple, easy-to-use blood-pressure cuffs for sale at drugstores and medical-supply stores. You just wrap the cuff around your arm, pump it up, and listen for the beeps. Usually, the beep starts to indicate your systolic, then stops to signal your diastolic.

Many people are finding that by monitoring their own blood pressure, watching their health progress, they are motivated to do the things the doctor has prescribed. Indeed, doctors are finding that just by monitoring the blood pressure, it often may go down. It makes people aware of their pressure and, half-unconsciously, they do more of the things that are good for their health.

Drugs: Are They Forever?

In the past, people who were given drugs for high blood pressure faced a lifetime of pill-taking. Now there's new hope that the pills may not be a permanent part of your life.

Dr. Rose Stamler, professor of community health and preventive medicine at Northwestern University, has been working with patients whose high blood pressure was first brought down to normal by Stepped Care. Then, gradually, she weaned these patients away from their pills.

A year and a half later, a great many of them were still normal, without drugs and without a change in diet. *Twice* as many, though, were able to stop pill-taking and stay normal if they also followed the doctor's orders to lose ten pounds, cut salt intake, increase exercise, and reduce alcohol to two drinks or less a day.

This is not something to try on your own. When your blood pressure is down to normal for a reasonable amount of time, it's something to discuss with your doctor.

In Addition to Drugs . . .

Along with a prescription for your pills, your doctor may have given you some of the same "orders" as Dr. Rose

Stamler gave to her patients. For more about diet and exercise, see Chapters 5, 6, 7, and 10.

Many doctors are just beginning to catch up with the new evidence on how psychological approaches can help physiological problems. As you take your medicine, you may want to ask your doctor about the relaxation methods discussed in Chapters 11 through 13 and about the anger-management technique in Chapter 14.

These nondrug therapies can help to make your drugs work better. For some people, they may make it possible to take a lower dose of the drugs and, after a while, if your doctor agrees, no dose at all.

5. Eating Smart: A Diet That Isn't Really a Diet

"You need to lose some weight . . ." the doctor tells you. For many people with hypertension, the numbers on the scale and the numbers on the sphygmomanometer go together. If you can bring the first one down, the second will follow.

Scientists have known since as early as 1925 that people who are overweight are five times more likely to have high blood pressure. Scientists also have observed that a drop in weight usually brings a drop in blood pressure.

Recently, at the University of California at Los Angeles School of Medicine, researchers had good news for people who weigh too much. All of the people in their study with high blood pressure managed to lower it significantly, to the normal range—even though most of them lost only 10 to 30 percent of what they needed to lose for an ideal weight. In other words, they got good-health results even without taking it *all* off.

There is growing evidence that for some people, those with milder hypertension, losing weight is all that's needed. With no pills, no sodium reduction, no other changes, some studies show that some people can get down to a normal pressure just by getting down to a more normal weight.

For other people, other changes are important. Some need to lose weight along with taking medication, as discussed in the previous chapter. Some need to lose weight along with watching their sodium, and we'll talk about that in Chapter 7.

For everyone with high blood pressure, extra pounds mean extra dangers. Hypertension and overweight both are high-risk factors for heart attacks. Lowering your weight lowers the threat to your health.

How, though, do you go about losing those extra pounds? Diet is something that's easier said than done. If you're overweight, chances are that you've tried it before. If you're still overweight, did you fail? Or did the diet fail?

In this chapter, we'll be talking about an eating plan that succeeds where others do not. Of course, you should talk to your doctor before going on any diet, but this is a program that's probably easier to stay on than anything else you may have tried. It's a diet that isn't really a diet.

Diet: A Four-Letter Word

For the sixty to eighty million Americans who are overweight, a diet is a curse. It is one of the dictionary's most unpleasant words. If you are on a typical diet, it means doing without. It means feeling deprived. It means wanting a brownie, a dish of ice cream, a glass of beer—whatever your favorite "forbidden" food is—and not having it.

Worst of all, most diets don't work. They are recipes for failure. Most people refuse to feel deprived forever, so a diet becomes something you go on—and then go off. A year after the diet, according to a number of studies, here is what happens:

- Almost all dieters have regained the weight they lost. If they have high blood pressure, that can mean they've also gained back the pressure they lowered.
- Some people have gained even more pounds than they lost on the diet.
- Only 3 to 5 percent have kept the weight off.

With results like that, it's no wonder that diets have become a growth industry, with a nonstop assembly line that produces a constant stream of new diets, new best-selling diet books, new spas or "fat farms," new promises.

Now there is a different eating plan—and with very different results. In a five-year follow-up survey of this program, more than half of the participants who responded—a remarkable 55 percent—had either kept off the weight they lost or had lost even more weight.

This record-breaking success rate—55 percent as compared to the usual 3 to 5 percent—was reported to physicians and nutritionists from all over the world at the Third International Conference on Obesity, held in Rome, Italy, in October of 1980. Among the people involved in carrying out the survey were Jules Hirsch, M.D., an internationally respected expert on obesity and inventor of "the fat-cell theory," and Joel Gurin, Ph.D., a leading medical researcher and coauthor of *The Dieter's Dilemma: Eating Less and Weighing More,* a book that explores the scientific theories of overweight.

A New Idea That Really Works

Green Mountain at Fox Run is the home of this creative, workable new approach to losing weight and keeping it off. A comfortable, unpretentious building, it is a former ski lodge set on a peaceful slope in Ludlow, Vermont. Today it is "an educational community for weight and health management."

They do not use the word "diet" at Green Mountain. There are no calories to count, no portions to weigh. There are no "good" and "bad" foods, no "legal" and "illegal" ones. There are no menus, setting out each day's breakfast, lunch, and dinner. (We'll be giving you some menus, but they are just suggestions, just illustrations of how well you can eat on this program.)

People learn new eating patterns at Green Mountain, but they do it by learning new thinking patterns. Many of them have tried everything else, from the Scarsdale to the Beverly Hills diets, from luxury spas to intestinal bypasses. Some of the people who come here have serious eating disorders, such as bulimia, a compulsive cycle of binge overeating and purging. Some need to lose one hundred pounds or more. In each class, there's always one woman who has already lost a hundred pounds. She has done it ten pounds at a time, over and over, one diet after another, the same ten pounds gained and lost and gained again.

Many of the people at Green Mountain are hard-core cases. What works for them is even more likely to work for the average person who is overweight. Generally, people spend four weeks at Green Mountain, learning to change their weight by changing their minds. The lessons they learn can be helpful to anyone who wants to lose some weight.

"If You Want It, Have It!"

A major reason why diets fail is guilt. Sooner or later, you grow weary of the diet's no-nos. In a moment when you feel stressed or lonely or unhappy, you yield to temptation. You comfort yourself with a brownie or some other forbidden food. Now you've gone off your diet. Do you now feel guilty, weak, a failure? Do you think, I blew it? Do you then go ahead and polish off the whole box of brownies?

That's the round-and-round of dieting, explains Thelma J. Wayler, nutritionist, former professor of nutrition education at Long Island University in New York and founder and director of Green Mountain. To Professor Wayler, the typical diet is a circle that looks like this:

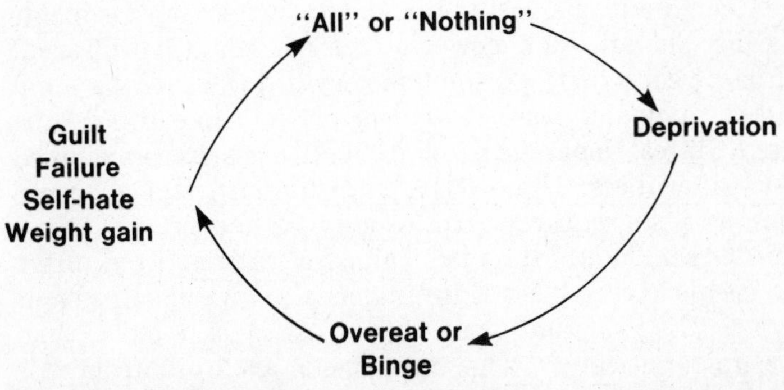

For most dieters, most diets begin by seeming like "nothing." There are no brownies—Professor Wayler's metaphor for cookies, cakes, ice cream, doughnuts, a cocktail or glass of beer, whatever your favorite forbidden foods are. That leads to feeling deprived . . . which leads to overeating . . . which leads to feeling guilty . . . which leads to more eating and more weight gain. If the choice is between "all" or "nothing," sooner or later most dieters choose "all."

The Green Mountain idea is to break that circle, to do away with feeling deprived and feeling guilty. Under the Green Mountain plan, it's not all or nothing, but something in between. You can have anything, but not *all* of anything. You can have everything, but not EVERYTHING.

That's the Option Plan, as they call it at Green Mountain. The theory states: If you want or need a brownie, you can have it, without feeling guilty. You deserve the brownie. You're a person, too.

Unlike the practice in other diet plans, the Option Plan is not an exchange, not a swap for some other foods on your daily menu. "If you exchange foods, you're exchanging nutrients, and unbalancing your diet," explains Professor Wayler. So this is "in addition to" whatever else you're eating.

"One brownie doesn't make you fat," says Professor Wayler. "Dieting makes you fat. Feeling guilty, so you eat the whole box of brownies, makes you fat."

How to "Eat Smart"

The Green Mountain eating plan begins where most sensible diets do. Though each new diet tries hard to be different from last year's diet, it seldom is very different. If it's not a fad diet, it usually is a rewriting of the same thing—the United States Department of Agriculture's Recommended Daily Allowances. These RDA's are the basics of good nutrition and the requirements for staying healthy.

The Green Mountain plan calls for eating three nutritious meals a day. "No skipping meals," warns Professor Wayler. "If you don't have breakfast, you'll more than make up for it later." The three meals are built from this basic framework:

Dairy products—2 servings, 170 calories
Animal products—2 servings, 530 calories
Fruits and vegetables—4 servings, 200 calories
Cereals and breads—2 servings, 100 calories
Fats—1 serving, 45 calories
"Ad libs"—coffee or tea, no cream, no sugar, no calories

That's a great deal of food, but it adds up to only 1,045 calories a day. Depending on your choices—whole milk versus low-fat milk, beef or pork versus chicken or fish—it could be somewhat more.

The Plank of Choice

If this looks like most diets, the difference is that most diets are "a tightrope," as Professor Wayler calls it, a strict and narrow line that's hard to stay on. Instead, she proposes "a plank of choice." The width of the plank is the difference between the calories you take in on the basic plan and the calories you burn up.

With moderate activity, you may be using up 1,800 calories a day. That means that if you have an "option"—a brownie for 146 calories, a slice of pizza for 236 calories, a glass of beer for 85 calories—you are still in "negative caloric balance," still losing weight.

What happens, though, if you have more than one option? Suppose you go out to a restaurant and have a drink before dinner, blue-cheese dressing on your salad, and chocolate mousse for dessert. That's not simply three options; it's "overeating," according to Professor Wayler. If you do enough of it, you may eat your way out of that nice, negative-calorie place. You probably won't lose weight that day.

"Thin people overeat, too," Professor Wayler points out. "You may be surprised to hear that, but a thin woman may go to a friend's wedding and eat too much. Then she wakes up the next morning and just gets on with her life. The overweight woman gets into trouble because she broods about it, feels guilty, and then eats some more."

Exercise Is the Key

As we discuss in Chapter 10, there is some evidence that exercise, just by itself, can lower blood pressure in some people. When you add exercise and diet together, you have a synergism; each makes the other work better, each multiplies the other's weight-loss and blood-pressure effects.

When you exercise, your metabolism changes. Your body's engine revs up, working at a higher, more efficient rate, burning more calories and so helping you to lose more weight. That improved metabolism happens when you do your exercise, and it continues to work for you between exercise periods.

The greatest benefits come with aerobic exercise, but even moderate and regular exercise can bring important changes. "If you simply take a walk for about twenty minutes in the morning and again in the evening," says Ann O'Connor, a Green Mountain nutritionist, "your metabolism can go up by a significant amount."

Exercise can also solve some of the great dilemmas of dieters. When you begin to eat a diet that's lower in calories, for example, your metabolism can go down after two or three days. That makes it harder to lose weight, but exercise can bring that metabolism back up.

It can also help to get you past your "set point." According to a new theory, each of us has a set point, a weight that the body yearns to be, a weight that it's very difficult to get past. Essentially, that set point is based on your metabolism and on the number of fat cells in your body. The number of those fat cells can't be reduced, but exercise and diet can make the cells themselves smaller. Exercise, by changing your metabolism, also makes it possible for your diet to continue working beyond your set point.

Exercise does something else that's important, something that changes the mind as well as the body. It gives you a positive, successful experience. Perhaps once you were huffing and puffing after walking a quarter of a mile, and now you can walk a full mile with ease. Perhaps once you could barely do five push-ups, and now you can do ten or fifteen.

Feeling good about yourself will help you to stay with your weight-loss plan. Becoming aware of your body will motivate you to shape it up. At Green Mountain, there are no glittering promises of how many pounds you will lose in how many days. People tend to lose more weight here than at other places. The success rate—taking it off and keeping it off—is higher than on other diets.

That happens because the Green Mountain program makes only this promise: *"You're going to learn to like yourself."* Exercise is a vital way of changing your body image and so your self-image.

Your Eating Patterns

If you're going to change any behavior, you first have to know what that behavior is. Many people aren't aware of how often they eat, how much they eat, even what they eat.

Yet the more aware you are of your eating patterns, the less "unaware" eating you'll do. The more you understand your food habits, the more you'll understand the feelings behind them. As Professor Wayler says, "It's the feelings, not the food, that make you fat."

A helpful Green Mountain tool is a Daily Food Diary, a record of what, where, and when you eat. You can begin such a diary with the sample chart on page 48. Then you can make additional pages, as you need them, by copying the chart on ordinary pieces of 8½-by-11-inch typing paper.

How to keep your diary:

Time—Under this heading, record the time you began and the time you ended each meal or snack. Record each eating event, even if it's a single gumdrop or a no-calorie cup of coffee.

Type and Amount of Intake—Record the kind of food or foods eaten and try to estimate how much—by weight, size of portion, or number of pieces.

Hunger—On a scale of 0 to 5, write down how hungry you felt just before eating.

Place—Write down the place where you ate the food—at home (which room), in a restaurant, at your desk, in your car, walking down the street, and so on.

DAILY FOOD DIARY

Day __________ Date __________ Your name __________

Time (Duration)	Type and Amount of Intake	Hunger 0 to 5	Place	Physical Position	Alone or with Others	Related Activity	Mood

Physical Position—As you ate, were you standing, sitting, lying down?

Alone or with Others—If eating alone, note that. If with others, write down who they were.

Related Activity—If you were doing anything else while eating—reading, watching television, talking on the phone—record that.

Mood—Write down how you felt just before eating—tense, depressed, happy, lonely, neutral.

If you keep this diary for a week or two, you'll see your personal pattern of eating. Some people will find that they eat only three meals a day, but that the portions are too large. Others will spot a pattern of constant snacking. Many will find that they're eating when they're not really hungry.

Changing Your Eating Patterns

Depending on what your food diary shows, try some or all of these good-eating ideas from Green Mountain:

- Slow down. Some overweight people manage to finish a complete meal in four minutes, but the faster you eat, the more you eat. You don't give yourself time to feel "full" or satisfied. So eat slower. Take smaller bites. Put your knife and fork down between bites.
- Use smaller plates, to make normal portions look larger.
- Whenever you're eating, even if it's just a snack, put the food on a plate and use a fork or spoon to eat it with. When people eat food out of a box or container, they're not thinking about how much they're eating, and usually they end up eating more than they'd planned.
- Always eat in the appropriate place—at the table. Don't eat standing up, at the refrigerator, or at the kitchen counter. Especially if you find you're doing a lot of eating in the TV room or the bedroom, try to restrict it to the kitchen table or the dining table.
- Plan ahead. Prepare a tray of snacks, the appropriate foods cut into appropriate portions. Then, when you're hungry for a snack, you won't be tempted to grab handfuls of just anything.

• Break up the pattern. If it's your habit to come home from work and head straight for the refrigerator, make a detour; change your clothes first. If you find that there are certain times of day when you feel stressed and so you overeat, try to deal with the stress in a different way. Schedule your exercise for those times. Or try the relaxation techniques in Chapters 11 and 13.

• If you find you're doing much of your overeating when you're alone, seek out companions for lunch and dinner. If you're eating just to have something to do, look for other ways to keep your hands busy—knitting, drawing, doodling, fingering worry beads, anything. Don't, though, take up smoking.

• For women, it's a good idea to plot out your menstrual cycle. You may see that the high and low mood swings of your monthly cycle are connected to the times you overeat. Or you may spot the days when you feel bloated, when your clothes suddenly don't fit, when you even weigh more. If you realize that it's only temporary, just a part of your menstrual cycle, it saves you from feeling discouraged about your diet and even giving up on it.

• Notice the kinds of foods you're eating. Some people tend toward soft foods—ice cream, puddings, cream soups; foods associated with emotional comfort, cuddling, and warmth. Other people will tend toward crunchy foods—nuts, chips, crackers; foods that let you get your teeth into them, a physical pleasure but sometimes a way of making noise to get rid of anger. If you can identify and understand what your feelings are, you can focus on those feelings rather than on the food.

Setting Your Priorities

Another helpful exercise from Green Mountain can assist you in getting your priorities in order. To begin, make a list of all your favorite foods, along with the amounts of each that you like to eat. Then make a second list of the things you want in life. On this list, you might put love, a better job, more friends, clothes that look well, good health, a new car, travel, and so on.

Compare the two lists. Now ask yourself, "If I have all the

things on the first list, what won't I be able to have on the second list?" Think about the trade-offs. You may, for example, be able to keep overeating and still buy a new car, but you may miss out on the new job, the wardrobe that fits and flatters, the good health and lower blood pressure.

For some people, there are advantages to being overweight. It's a protective wall against having to compete in love, work, or friendships. It's a built-in excuse when something goes wrong. "When you decide that the rewards of being thinner are greater than the rewards of being fatter," says Professor Wayler, "then you'll be thinner."

Learning to Like Yourself

This is the real secret of this program, learning to feel good about yourself. Most diets keep you from doing that, because they make you feel deprived, unworthy of the treats other people are enjoying. Or they treat you like a child. It is demeaning to be told what to eat and when, every meal, day in and day out.

On this plan, you're an adult, capable of making your own responsible choices. You're in control of your own life, the giant step to being in control of your own weight—and blood pressure.

Begin today to take the step—with our next chapter on cooking tips, suggested menus, and recipes.

6. Cooking Smart

Hang on to your old cookbooks. Don't toss away your favorite recipes. All it takes are a few changes, to turn almost any recipe into a "smart" recipe.

That means low in calories. It also means low in some of the other things that can be connected to high blood pressure—low in salt, low in cholesterol, low in fat.

To show you how varied and flavorful and filling a "diet" can be, we asked the nutritionists at Green Mountain to prepare some sample menus. They're here to start you thinking about your own menus. So you can follow them as closely or as loosely as you like. You can switch one day with any other. You can trade one lunch or dinner with another. Just bear in mind the Recommended Daily Allowances for good nutrition, as listed on page 45.

The menus that follow add up like this:

Average daily calories—1,000 (without optional evening snack)
Average daily sodium—1,251 mg. or 1.25 grams
Average daily cholesterol—246.7 mg.
Average percentage of calories as fat—26 percent

A Guide to Good Eating

In the menus that follow, you'll find an asterisk(*) next to each dish for which we'll be giving you cooking tips later in this chapter, so you can see how easy it is to modify almost any recipe. You'll find a double asterisk (**) next to each dish for which we'll be giving you the recipe, so you can see how it's done. As you'll discover, there's no mystery at all to adapting your favorite foods to this eating program.

Note that each meal ends with a beverage. This can be coffee (regular or decaffeinated) or tea (hot or iced). In addition, you are urged to drink two glasses of skim milk each day, but it's your choice as to what time you have them.

Also note that when the menu calls for salad, you may use your favorite dressing, one tablespoon, once a day. At other times, try our "Zero" Salad Dressing**. Or try a simple sprinkling of vinegar or lemon juice.

Sunday

BREAKFAST

Orange juice (4 oz.)
or
Prune juice (3 oz.)
or
Fresh orange (1 med.)
*Blueberry muffin**
or
Cream of Wheat cereal (½ cup)
or
Nonsweetened cold cereal (¾ cup)
or
Toast (1 slice, whole wheat or rye) with 2 oz. low-fat cottage cheese
Beverage

LUNCH

*Chicken or Sirloin Kabobs** (2 oz.) with rice (4 oz.)*

Onion/tomato wedge/green pepper salad
or
Choose your own salad of
tuna or low-fat cottage cheese or
hard-boiled egg—with your favorite
salad dressing (1 tbs.) or
*"Zero" Salad Dressing***
Fruit gelatin
Beverage

DINNER

*Eggplant Parmigiana***
Spinach salad with dressing
Fresh fruit bowl
Beverage

Monday

BREAKFAST

Orange juice (4 oz.)
or
Prune juice (3 oz.)
or
Banana (½)
Cold cereal (¾ cup)
or
Oatmeal (½ cup)
or
Toast (1 slice, whole wheat or
rye) with peanut butter (1 tsp. unsalted)
Beverage

LUNCH

Cheese pizza (2 slices)*
Green salad with dressing
Fresh fruit
Beverage

DINNER

Baked fresh fish (4 oz.)
Steamed summer squash (½ cup)

Marinated cucumber salad
Vanilla ice cream (½ cup)
Beverage

Tuesday

BREAKFAST

Orange juice (4 oz.)
  or
Prune juice (3 oz.)
  or
Grapefruit juice (4 oz.)
Cold cereal (¾ cup)
  or
Wheatena (½ cup)
  or
Toast (1 slice) with
  low-fat cottage cheese (2 oz.)
Beverage

LUNCH

*Onion soup**
  with cheese and croutons
Tossed salad with dressing
Fresh fruit salad
Beverage

DINNER

Grilled liver (3 oz.)
  and onions
Fresh corn (½ ear)
*First Frost***
Beverage

Wednesday

BREAKFAST

Orange juice (4 oz.)
  or

Prune juice (3 oz.)
or
Fresh grapefruit (½)
Poached egg (1) on
toast (1 slice, whole wheat or rye)
or
Cream of Wheat (½ cup)
or
Cold cereal (¾ cup)
Beverage

LUNCH

Make-your-own salad
with a choice of:
Mixed greens
Cherry tomatoes
Grated carrot
Cauliflower or broccoli flowerets
Cucumber slices
Green pepper rings
Mushroom slices
plus
Grated cheeses—cheddar or part-skim mozzarella
plus
Kidney beans
Garbanzo beans
plus
Croutons (toast and cut up 1 slice of bread)
plus
Salad dressing—chunky blue cheese, creamy Italian, or Thousand Island

DINNER

Roast chicken pieces (1 breast or 1 leg and thigh, 4 oz.)
*Oven-Browned Potato Spears***
Green salad with dressing
Fresh fruit
Beverage

Thursday

BREAKFAST

Orange juice (4 oz.)
or
Prune juice (3 oz.)
or
*Applesauce***
(⅓ cup)
Oatmeal (½ cup)
or
Cold cereal (¾ cup)
or
Toast (1 slice) with
low-fat cottage cheese (2 oz.)
Beverage

LUNCH

*Mushroom omelette**
Bread (1 thin slice)
or
Melba toast (2 slices)
*Cold Vegetable Salad***
Pineapple (2 slices packed in juice)
Beverage

DINNER

Veal patties (4 oz.) with
mushroom, onion, and green pepper
Romaine salad with dressing
*Baked Apple***
Beverage

Friday

BREAKFAST

Orange juice (4 oz.)
or
Prune juice (3 oz.)
or

Pineapple juice (4 oz.)
*Bran muffin**
or
Cream of Rice (½ cup)
or
Cold cereal (¾ cup)
or
Toast (1 slice) with
cheddar cheese (¾ oz.)
Beverage

LUNCH

Tuna and potato salad
(2 oz. tuna and 4 oz. potato salad)
Coffee ice cream (½ cup)
Beverage

DINNER

*Zucchini Tofu Lasagna***
Spinach salad with dressing
Sliced fresh orange, garnished with mint
Beverage

Saturday

BREAKFAST

Orange juice (4 oz.)
or
Prune juice (3 oz.)
or
Tomato juice (4 oz.)
Pancakes with blueberry sauce
or
Wheatena (½ cup)
or
Cold cereal (¾ cup)
or
Toast (1 slice) with
low-fat cottage cheese (2 oz.)
Beverage

LUNCH

Beef taco
(2 oz. beef, 1 taco shell with lettuce, tomato, onion)
Fresh fruit
Beverage

DINNER

*Pasta Primavera***
Lettuce-wedge salad with dressing
*Baked Pear Halves***
Beverage

Suggestions for an Evening Snack (*Optional*)
Fresh fruit (1 piece)
or
Cheese (such as cheddar, 1 oz.) with melba toast (2 slices)
or
Low-fat cottage cheese (2 oz.) with melba toast (2 slices)
or
Peanut butter (2 tsp.) with melba toast (2 slices)
or
Unsalted peanuts (1 oz.)
Beverage

Cooking Tips and Techniques

• At first, as you cut back on fats and on salt, your foods will taste different. For many people, they will seem to be bland and to have no taste at all. Your taste buds have been trained to like certain flavors, but after a week or so, those taste buds will be reeducated. Now you'll begin to savor the real flavors of the foods themselves. You'll discover new tastes that were hidden by your old ways of cooking. So be patient on those first few no-taste days.

• On this plan, there's no need to cook one meal for yourself and another for the rest of the family. These menus are healthy, nutritious, and satisfying for anyone. People who are watching their weight or their blood pressure should stay with the portions we've suggested. People who don't need to worry about those things can help themselves to "seconds."

• In baking almost anything, you can reduce the amount of sugar that the recipe calls for by one-third, without hurting the recipe. If the recipe calls for salt, omit it. Except for yeast-raised baked products, salt serves no function other than pleasing taste buds that are accustomed to it.

• More baking tips: In place of shortening or solid fats, use vegetable oils; sunflower, soybean, or safflower are best. To cut down the amount of cholesterol, discard one of the egg yolks called for in your recipe and replace it with one tablespoon of vegetable oil. Use a vegetable spray product to "grease" your baking pans. Modified in this way, your favorite recipe for muffins, such as blueberry or bran, can make a complete breakfast, along with juice or fruit and a beverage.

• Pizza is a no-no on most diets, but even two slices of cheese pizza can be "smart" eating. Use any recipe you like for the pizza dough. If it includes any salt, sugar, or fat, these may be safely omitted, say the Green Mountain experts. For the topping, use tomato sauce and a mixture of grated, part-skim mozzarella and provolone cheeses.

• For onion soup or any other soup, begin with our recipe for low-calorie, salt-free beef or chicken stock. To sauté the onions or other vegetables that your favorite recipe calls for, spray a hot pan with a vegetable spray product and add several tablespoons of the stock. This is the method that Green Mountain nutritionists recommend for all "sautéing." Try omitting any oil in your soup recipes. Use skim or low-fat milk in "cream" soups. A little wine goes a long way, so if your recipe calls for wine, decrease the amount. Be sure to use table wines rather than the "cooking wines" that contain added salt.

• Omelettes can be a quick and tasty meal. Try discarding one yolk per two eggs, to decrease the cholesterol content by half. For a filling, use low-fat cheeses (ricotta, cottage, part-skim mozzarella), herbs, and/or "sautéed" mushrooms or other vegetables.

• Though almost any recipe can be modified, there are some recipes that insist on being themselves. Southern fried chicken calls for deep-frying, though some people enjoy the taste of oven-fried. Beef strogonoff demands sour cream, though some people substitute yogurt and like the different taste. There will be a recipe or two that you want to use but that you can't transform into a "smart" recipe. "If you want it, have it as an option," says Professor Wayler. Just try not to have it too often, and pay attention to the size of the portion.

• Experiment with herbs and spices. They are all goodness and flavor, with no sodium, no cholesterol, no fat, no calories. They add taste and enhance the natural flavors of food. For more about the flavor adventures of herbs and spices, see Chapter 7 for a guide on which ones go best with which foods.

• In Chapter 7, on "Shaking the Salt Habit," the do-it-yourself menu plan and a number of the suggested tips and techniques can be helpful for a weight-loss program as well as for a lower-salt diet.

"Smart" Recipes

CHICKEN OR SIRLOIN KABOBS

¼ cup soy sauce
¾ cup salt-free broth or water
3 tablespoons vinegar
8 green pepper wedges
8 onion wedges
½ to ¾ pound boned chicken breasts or flank steak, cut into 8 strips
8 cherry tomatoes
8 mushrooms

1. Combine the soy sauce, broth (or water), and vinegar, to make the marinade.
2. Blanch the green peppers and onions.
3. For each kabob, place on a skewer 2 beef or chicken strips and 2 of each vegetable.
4. Set kabobs in a shallow pan and pour the marinade over them. Marinate for at least one hour, turning occasionally.

5. Remove kabobs from marinade, place on a flat cookie sheet, and bake at 400° F for 20 to 25 minutes, until done.

Serve with rice.

Yield: 4 servings.

EGGPLANT PARMIGIANA

2 large eggplants
1 to 1½ quarts tomato sauce (plain or flavored with your favorite herbs and spices)
1¼ pounds part-skim mozzarella cheese, thinly sliced
Parmesan cheese

1. Slice the eggplants into thin circles (⅓ to ¼ inches thick) or make thin lengthwise slices.
2. Broil lightly on both sides.
3. Cover the bottom of a 9-by-13-inch pan with a layer of the tomato sauce. Then make a layer of eggplant, a layer of mozzarella cheese slices, a layer of sauce. Continue to alternate the layers, ending with a top layer of sauce.
4. Bake, covered, at 325° F for about one hour. Remove from oven and sprinkle with Parmesan cheese. When cooled, cut into 12 squares. This dish is best if allowed to sit several hours or overnight, then rewarmed before serving. (This dish lends itself especially well to freezing—in family or individual portions—to use for later no-fuss meals.)

Yield: 12 servings. Use as needed and freeze remainder.

ZUCCHINI TOFU LASAGNA

3 to 3½ pounds zucchini squash
3 pounds tofu
1 to 1½ quarts tomato sauce (plain or flavored with your favorite herbs and spices)
Parmesan cheese

1. Cut the zucchini into thin slices (⅓ to ¼ inches thick).
2. Broil lightly on both sides.
3. Make thin slices (¼ inch thick) of the tofu.
4. In a 9-by-13-inch pan, spread enough sauce to cover the bot-

tom. Then add alternating layers of zucchini, tofu, and sauce. Continue to alternate the layers, ending with a top layer of sauce.

5. Bake, covered, at 325 °F for about one hour. Remove from oven and sprinkle with Parmesan cheese. Let cool slightly and cut into 12 squares. This dish is best if allowed to sit for a few hours or overnight, then rewarmed before serving. (Another dish that freezes very well, in family or individual portions. Keep on hand for days when there's no time to cook.)

Yield: 12 servings. Use as needed and freeze remainder.

PASTA PRIMAVERA

Following our cooking tips and techniques, you can modify any "primavera" recipe. Or follow these easy steps:

1. Steam a good variety of vegetables, whatever is in season or to your taste.
2. When pasta is cooked and drained, toss pasta and vegetables together.
3. Portion into individual bowls and sprinkle generously with Parmesan cheese.

COLD VEGETABLE SALAD

½ cup assorted cooked vegetables per serving
Yogurt Dressing (see below)

1. Use any leftover cooked vegetables that you have on hand. Or blanch a combination of vegetables—carrots, corn, and peas, for example, or broccoli, cauliflower, and carrots.
2. Mix chilled vegetables with yogurt dressing.
3. Chill. Then, for each serving, arrange ½ cup of mixture on a bed of lettuce.

YOGURT DRESSING

1 cup plain, low-fat yogurt
1 tablespoon lemon juice
1 cup cucumber, finely chopped
¼ teaspoon garlic powder
1 teaspoon dill

1. Combine all ingredients and mix well.
2. Use as needed.
3. Store, covered, in refrigerator.

Yield: 2 cups.

"ZERO" SALAD DRESSING

1 quart tomato juice
1/6 cup lemon juice
2 teaspoons garlic powder
2 teaspoons dry mustard
5 teaspoons minced onion
6 teaspoons Worcestershire sauce
2 teaspoons horseradish
Dash of sugar or sugar substitute

1. Combine all ingredients and mix well.
2. Use as needed. Stir well before using.
3. Store, covered, in refrigerator.

Yield: One quart.

SWEET 'N' SOUR DRESSING

1 cup water
2 cups red wine or apple cider vinegar
1 teaspoon or less sugar substitute

1. Combine ingredients and mix well. Use 1 teaspoon or less of the sugar substitute, to suit your taste.
2. Use as needed on salads.
3. Store, covered, in refrigerator.

Yield: 3 cups.

OVEN-BROWNED POTATO SPEARS

For each serving, use one medium potato:

1. Wash skin well but do not peel.
2. Cut into spears, chunky pieces such as steak fries.
3. They can be browned by themselves but are best if added to the pan in which you are roasting chicken or other meats.
4. They should bake for about one hour at medium heat.
5. Drain on a paper towel before serving.

CHICKEN OR BEEF STOCK (FOR SOUPS AND "SAUTÉING")

8 pounds chicken or beef bones and parts (chicken neck, back, giblets)
5 quarts water
½ pound onions, diced
¼ pound carrots, diced
¼ pound celery, diced
Herbs and spices to taste (bay leaf, peppercorns, bouquet garni)

1. Place bones and parts in stockpot and add water. (If you are making less stock than this recipe calls for, or more stock, simply add enough cold water to cover bones.)
2. Add vegetables and herbs and spices.
3. Bring to a boil, then reduce heat to low. Simmer chicken stock for 2 to 4 hours; beef stock for 6 to 8 hours. The longer the stock simmers, the stronger it will be.
4. From time to time, as the stock simmers, skim off the fatty film that forms on top.
5. When done, strain stock, using a strainer or cheesecloth.
6. When stock has cooled to room temperature, cover, tape on a label with the date, then place in the refrigerator. This stock should keep about one week in the refrigerator, and much longer in your freezer.
7. When the stock has chilled in the refrigerator, the fat will form a top layer or crust. Remove this before using, to make the stock fat-free.
8. Try freezing your own bouillon cubes. Pour stock into an ice-cube tray and freeze. Use the cubes as you need them, for soup-making or "sautéing."

Yield: 4 quarts. (If you are making less stock than this recipe calls for, yield will be about three-fourths of amount with water added.)

FIRST FROST

1. Core but do not peel one apple per serving.
2. Grate the apple.

3. Place in a sherbet glass or wine goblet. Pour in enough orange juice to cover the grated apple.
4. Garnish with a twist of orange peel.
5. Serve chilled.

APPLESAUCE

1. Core and slice 6 tart apples—or as many apples for the amount of applesauce you want to make.
2. If you're going to be using a food mill, leave the peels on, for extra flavor and color. If not, peel the apples.
3. Place sliced apples in a saucepan and add enough apple juice to cover.
4. Simmer over low heat for 20 minutes or until the apples are very soft.
5. Put through the food mill, or stir well by hand.
6. Add cinnamon and nutmeg to taste.

Yield: 4 servings.

BAKED APPLE

1. Core but do not peel one apple per serving.
2. Place in baking dish and add apple juice or diet ginger ale or other soda.
3. Bake 15 to 20 minutes in moderate oven.

BAKED PEAR HALVES

Fresh pears (one whole one per serving)
or
Canned pear halves, water or juice packed (2 halves per serving)
½ teaspoon vanilla extract
Dash of lemon juice
Sugar substitute
Slice of lemon for garnish

1. If using fresh pears, peel, core, and cut in half. Then pour 2 cups of water into a saucepan. If using canned pears, pour liquid from can into saucepan and add enough water to make 2 cups of liquid.

2. To the liquid, add vanilla extract, dash of lemon juice, and dash of sugar substitute. Heat to boiling, then simmer for 20 minutes to reduce liquid.

3. Add pear halves. Cover and cook over low heat for 30 minutes.

4. Serve 2 halves in a dessert dish, garnished with a slice of lemon.

7. Shaking the Salt Habit

"Cut down on salt." If you have high blood pressure, you've probably heard that from your doctor—and more than once. To most doctors, salt is a major culprit in this disease, and using less of it is a major cure.

If the doctor has prescribed "less salt" for you, how do you go about following that prescription? How low is a low-salt diet?

The good news is that it's not as low as it once was. Doctors used to put patients on severe salt restrictions. They wanted to drastically lower the amount of sodium (the ingredient in salt—or sodium chloride—that's connected to high blood pressure). The average person may be taking in 8 to 10 grams (or 8,000 to 10,000 milligrams) of sodium a day. People with high blood pressure were being asked to cut back to 1 gram or less a day.

"It was so radical as not to be practical," reports Dr. Thomas G. Pickering of the Hypertension Center of The New York Hospital–Cornell Medical Center. People couldn't stay on that severe a diet. Sooner or later, and mostly sooner, they would give up on it.

Today, most doctors are prescribing diets that are moderately low in sodium—1½ to 2 grams a day—or moderate in sodium—2 to 3 grams a day, except for some people with severe hypertension. People can eat well on this milder regime, and so they are more likely to stay with it.

Even with a milder sodium reduction, there's growing evidence that that's enough to lower the blood pressure. For some people, lowering the salt intake is the only prescription they may get. For others, it's in addition to taking medication, losing weight, or whatever else the doctor has advised.

The problem with sodium is that it is everywhere. It is a mineral that's found in nearly all the plants and animals we use as food. It's obvious in foods that taste salty, but it can surprise you. It can be there even when you don't taste it, when the food seems sweet.

You have to educate yourself. It may mean shopping for different foods, or cooking your familiar dishes in new but still tasty ways. Before your next trip to the supermarket, check your shopping list against the sodium list on page 70.

A Personal Plan for Good Eating

Now that you know which foods are high in sodium and which are better choices, you can begin to think about what you want to put on your plate. The menus listed in Chapter 6 are not only low in calories but low in sodium. They're a good starting point, chock-full of ideas on how tasty and balanced meals can be put together.

The best diet of all, though, is the one you're going to stay on. That means the one you're going to enjoy eating. Each of us has food prejudices and preferences. There are things we enjoy eating and cuisines we like above all others. You can follow those preferences by doing-it-yourself.

With the following chart, you can make a personal eating plan. Within limits—but wide limits—the choices are yours to make, and that's a happy way to start off on any diet. As always, though, check with your doctor first.

This program is for people who've been told to use mild sodium restriction, but it allows for menus that the whole

TABLE 1. Your Guide to the Sodium Content of Various Foods*

	Emphasize These (Foods LOW in sodium; less than 100 mg. per serving)	*Use in Moderation* (Foods MEDIUM in sodium; 100–400 mg. per serving)	*Beware of These* (Foods HIGH in sodium; over 400 mg. per serving)
SPICES, SAUCES, & CONDIMENTS	Unsalted seasonings: Basil Bay leaf Cinnamon Cloves Curry Dill Dry mustard Oregano Paprika Pepper Thyme Bitters Garlic (fresh or powdered) Mint Onion (fresh or powdered) Parsley Tabasco sauce Tomato (fresh or paste) Vanilla Vinegar Most salt substitutes (check with your doctor)	Lightly salted seasonings: Barbecue sauces Ketchup Chili sauce Gravies Mayonnaise Mustard Prepared salad dressings Steak sauce Tomato puree or sauce Worcestershire sauce	Salt Highly salted seasonings: Bouillon Lemon-pepper marinade Salted meat tenderizers Salt/salt substitute mixtures Salted spices (garlic salt, onion salt, seasoned salt) Soy sauce Teriyaki sauce

GRAINS & CEREALS	Unsalted grain products: Low-sodium breads & crackers Flour Hot cereals (except instant) Matzo Noodles Puffed rice or wheat Rice Shredded Wheat Corn tortillas Unsalted popcorn Whole grains Baked products made without salt, baking powder, or baking soda	Grain products made with small amounts of salt, baking powder, or baking soda: Bread & rolls Dry cereals Biscuits & muffins Cakes Cookies Pastries Pies Doughnuts Pancakes & waffles (Baking soda and baking powder contain sodium. Avoid using large amounts. Baked products made using yeast are good alternatives.)	Highly salted grain products: Commercially prepared spaghetti & pasta dishes Instant hot cereals Pretzels Salted crackers & chips Salted popcorn
VEGETABLES & FRUITS	Fruits Fruit juices Unsalted vegetables (except as noted)	Beet greens Celery Chard Lightly salted vegetables Canned vegetables Frozen lima beans Frozen peas	Highly salted vegetables: All pickled vegetables Olives & pickles Sauerkraut Vegetable juices Vegetables with seasoned sauces

TABLE 1. Your Guide to the Sodium Content of Various Foods* (continued)

	Emphasize These (Foods LOW in sodium; less than 100 mg. per serving)	*Use in Moderation* (Foods MEDIUM in sodium; 100–400 mg. per serving)	*Beware of These* (Foods HIGH in sodium; over 400 mg. per serving)
FISH, POULTRY, MEAT, & OTHER MAIN DISHES	Fresh meat prepared without salt: Beef Veal Fish Lamb Poultry Pork Dried beans cooked without salt or salt pork Eggs Unsalted nuts (To control fat, choose lean meats, poultry, fish, and beans.)	Fresh shellfish Salted nuts Salted peanut butter	Smoked, cured, or pickled products: Bacon Corned beef Dried meat or fish Ham Luncheon meats Sausages & frankfurters Fish or meat canned with salt Frozen dinners Most commercially prepared entrées Packaged or canned soups
DAIRY PRODUCTS	Cream cheese Gruyère cheese Ricotta cheese Swiss cheese Unsalted cheese Cream	Milk Buttermilk Cheese (except as noted) Custard Ice cream Pudding	American cheese Blue cheese Cottage cheese Parmesan cheese Roquefort cheese Processed cheese products

	Unsalted butter or margarine Sherbet (To control fat, choose low-fat dairy products, limit butter, margarine, and cream.)	Salted butter & margarine Yogurt	
BEVERAGES	Beer, liquor, & wine (moderation advised) Carbonated beverages Coffee & tea Most mineral waters (check with supplier)	Milk Buttermilk	

TABLE 2. For Mild Sodium Restriction*
Follow This Chart Every Day

What to Have Each Day—and How Much	*Use*	*Things to Know*	*Do Not Use*
Milk 2 glasses (Each glass contains about 170 calories)	Regular (whole) milk, evaporated milk, skim milk, buttermilk, reconstituted powdered milk. If you use skim milk, buttermilk, or powdered milk, you may add extra fat to your diet to make up for the fat that has been removed from the milk. For each glass, add 2 servings of fat. *Substitutes* for not more than 1 glass of milk a day: 2 ounces of meat, poultry, or fish; or 6 ounces of plain yogurt (¾ of a cup).	A glass of milk = 1 cup or 8 ounces A half cup of evaporated milk counts as a glass of milk. With powdered milk, follow the directions on the box for making 1 cup.	Because of the extra calories they contain, avoid ice cream, sherbet, malted milk, milk shakes, instant cocoa mixes, chocolate milk, condensed milk, and all other kinds of milk and fountain drinks.

Meat, Poultry, & Fish 5 ounces, cooked (Each ounce contains about 75 calories.)	Fresh, frozen, or canned meat or poultry: any kind except those listed in the last column. Fish or shellfish (fresh, frozen, or canned): any kind except those listed in the last column. *Substitutes* for 1 ounce of meat, poultry, or fish: an egg; ¼ cup of lightly salted cottage cheese; 1 ounce natural American cheddar or Swiss cheese; 2 tablespoons low-sodium dietetic peanut butter.	An average serving of meat or poultry is 3 ounces. (Allow an extra ounce or two for shrinkage, bone, and fat when you shop.) Examples of 3-ounce servings: 1 pork chop; 2 rib lamb chops; half breast or leg and thigh of 3-pound chicken; 2 meat patties, 2 inches across and ½ inch thick; 2 thin slices of roast beef, each 3 by 3 by ¼ inches.	Salty or smoked meat (bacon, bologna, chipped or corned beef, frankfurters, ham, luncheon meats, salt pork, sausage, smoked tongue) Salty or smoked fish (anchovies, caviar, salted cod, herring, sardines, etc.) Processed cheese or cheese spreads unless low-sodium dietetic; cheeses such as Roquefort, Camembert, or Gorgonzola. Regular peanut butter.
Vegetables At least 3 servings (Each starchy vegetable contains about 70 calories; other vegetables contain from 5 to 35 calories.)	Any vegetables except those listed in the last column. Fresh or frozen are best, since canned vegetables generally have salt added.	Count as a serving: about ½ cup of vegetable.	Sauerkraut, pickles, or other vegetables prepared in brine or heavily salted.

TABLE 2. For Mild Sodium Restriction* (continued)
Follow This Chart Every Day

What to Have Each Day—and How Much	*Use*	*Things to Know*	*Do Not Use*
Fruit 4 servings (Each serving contains about 40 calories.)	Any kind of fruit or fruit juice—fresh, frozen, canned, or dried—if sugar has not already been added.	The size of serving varies, depending on the fruit and the calories. Examples: 1 small apple: ½ cup fruit cup; 2 medium plums; 1 cup strawberries; 1 cup watermelon. If you do want sweetened fruit or fruit juice, add an allowed sugar substitute or the amount of sugar, honey, etc., allowed under "And . . . take your choice."	Because of the extra calories they contain, do not use: fruits canned or frozen in sugar syrup.
Breads, Cereals, etc. 7 servings (Each serving contains about 70 calories.)	Breads, rolls, and lightly salted crackers; lightly salted cereals; dry cereals; matzo; melba toast; macaroni, noodles, spaghetti, rice, barley; lightly salted popcorn; flour.	Count as a serving: 1 slice bread; 1 roll or muffin; 4 crackers or pieces of melba toast; ½ cup cooked cereal; ¾ cup dry cereal; ½ cup cooked noodles, rice, etc.; 1½ cups	Bread and rolls with salt topping; regular salted popcorn, potato chips, corn chips, pretzels, etc. Because of the extra calories they contain, avoid sugar-coated ce-

	Substitute for a serving of bread or cereal: a starchy vegetable.	popcorn, 2½ tablespoons flour	reals, pastries, cakes, sweet rolls, cookies
Fat 4 servings (Each serving contains about 45 calories.)	Butter or margarine; cooking fat or oil; French dressing; mayonnaise; heavy or light cream; unsalted nuts; avocado.	Count as a serving: 1 level teaspoon (or small pat) butter, margarine, fat, oil, or mayonnaise; 1 tablespoon heavy cream (sweet or sour); 2 tablespoons light cream; 1 tablespoon French dressing; 6 small nuts; ⅛ of a 4-inch avocado.	Bacon or bacon fat; salt pork; olives; salted nuts; party spreads and dips and other heavily salted snack foods, such as potato chips and sticks, crackers, etc.
And . . . Take Your Choice Choose 2 (Each choice contains about 75 calories.)	Each of these is 1 choice: 1 serving of bread, cereal, or starchy vegetable; 2 servings of fat; 4 teaspoons of sugar, honey, syrup, molasses, jelly, jam, or marmalade; candy made without salted nuts (75 calories worth).	These choices are intended to give you more freedom in planning your day's meals. They are part of your diet, to be included every day. You may split these choices if you wish. For example, 1 serving of fruit and 2 teaspoons of sugar could make 1 choice.	

TABLE 2. For Mild Sodium Restriction* (continued)
Follow This Chart Every Day

What to Have Each Day—and How Much	*Use*	*Things to Know*	*Do Not Use*
Miscellaneous	Use as desired: coffee, tea, coffee substitutes, sugar substitutes, lemons or limes, gelatin, vinegar, cream of tartar, baking powder and baking soda (for baking only), yeast.	When listed on food labels, the words "soda" or "sodium" or the symbol "Na" tell you that the product contains sodium.	Canned soups or stews; commercial bouillon cubes, powders, or liquids. These foods contain extra calories you may want to avoid: baking chocolate, cocoa and cocoa mixes, fruit-flavored beverage mixes, sugar-sweetened soft drinks, gelatin desserts, custards and puddings; cornstarch, cornmeal, tapioca.

family will enjoy. It is based on eating 1,800 calories a day. If your doctor has advised you to have fewer calories than that, or more calories, here's how to adapt the program:

Changes for 1,200 calories: For "Milk," use skim milk, buttermilk, or powdered milk only, and do not add the extra fat that's allowed under 1,800 calories. You may substitute one ounce of meat, poultry, or fish for one glass of milk a day. For "Breads," use four servings instead of seven. For "Fats," use no servings, unless you want to use one serving as a "choice."

Under "And . . . Take Your Choice," take one choice instead of two.

Changes for unrestricted calories: Extra servings: You may have extra servings of any allowed food. Additional foods: You may have any of the foods that are ruled out on the chart because of the calories. You may also have alcoholic beverages (with your doctor's permission).

Tips, Tricks, and Techniques for Success

In Chapter 5, talking about how to lower your blood pressure by lowering your weight, we discussed the Green Mountain idea of the Option Plan. As this theory goes: If you want it, have it. The idea is to allow yourself the treat you yearn for, so that you avoid the vicious cycle of typical diets—feeling deprived, feeling guilty, overeating, giving up on the diet.

Can this work on an eating plan where you're watching your salt? On this program, the foods that are generally off limits because of calories could be used as "options" or "double choices." For the foods that are banned because of their sodium content, the American Heart Association advises, "Don't make a habit of making exceptions."

At the Hypertension Center of The New York Hospital, Beatrice Di Fabio, R.D. (Registered Dietitian), has been working with the physicians on major diet-research studies and has been counseling individual patients on their personal eating programs. As she advises, "It's better to follow your diet six days a week and have a favorite food on the seventh day than not to follow your diet at all. Your body doesn't respond minute by minute but on the longer term.

So one bad day, one infraction of the rules, doesn't change your ongoing effort.

"Learn to trade off," she urges. "If you have something like pizza for lunch one day a week, learn to eliminate other salt or other fat for the rest of that day."

Other ideas from dietitian Di Fabio:

• American industry is on your side. Each month, an average of four new products appears on the supermarket shelves, either sodium-free or low in sodium. They range, literally, from soup to nuts. There now are low-sodium main dishes and desserts, sauces and canned vegetables, sodas and bouillon cubes, unsalted nuts and unsalted potato chips. (You may find that unsalted chips are crisper and crunchier than the regular kind, because salt is moisture-loving.) Make it a habit to read the labels. If the products contain potassium chloride, ask your doctor about that. Generally, the salt substitutes that are now available contain potassium chloride, and it's wise to check with your doctor on how much of that to be using.

• When you begin a lower-salt diet, food may taste bland. Be reassured that the "no-taste" syndrome will pass. For some people, the taste threshold will change in just a few days, and they'll begin to savor the real and natural flavors of foods. For other people, the change may take a couple of weeks.

• Experiment with the condiments that "mimic" a salt taste, especially lemon juice or vinegar.

• When you broil or pan-fry foods, try deglazing the pan, a favorite technique of French chefs. Remove the meat or fish you've been broiling or frying and pour in some water, a bit of orange juice or lemon juice, or a splash of wine. Stir over high heat until the browned bits and juices are reconstituted and thickened. Pour this concentrated flavor over your meat or fish.

• You can dine out and still stay on your diet. Most restaurants will cooperate with you, although, alas, the more expensive the restaurant, the easier it is. Fast-food restaurants can be a problem. In any restaurant, it's safest to stay with food in its most natural, most recognizable, most undisguised and unsauced form. For example, baked potatoes rather than mashed, since restaurants often prepare mashed potatoes from a dehydrated and highly salted product. It's simple to order broiled meats or fish and ask for no gravy. With salad, you can ask for the cruets of oil and vinegar and fix your own dressing.

• Toss your salad. Then toss it again. The more you toss a salad, the less dressing you need to use for the same good taste.

• Treat yourself to one tablespoon of grated Parmesan cheese a day. Yes, it's high in calories (23 of them) and sodium (93 mg.). If you're not on severe sodium restriction, this tablespoon can go a long way. A bit of it can have a high-flavor reward sprinkled on vegetables; on salad, instead of a lot of dressing; on fish when you're broiling it; or on unsalted and unbuttered popcorn.

• If your physician advised a very low sodium diet, at home or in a restaurant, try an order of French fries (if calories don't matter) or a plain baked potato as a substitute for regular salted bread.

A New World of Tastes

Think positively. Concentrate on the new tastes you can discover, instead of the old salt taste that you're doing without. If that sounds Pollyannaish, it's also true. There are many, many ways to enhance the natural flavors of food.

Instead of salt in your salt shaker, for example, try the American Heart Association's recipe for an "herb shaker" to use in the kitchen and at the table. Combine one-half teaspoon of cayenne pepper, one tablespoon of garlic powder, and one teaspoon of each of the following ground seasonings: basil, marjoram, thyme, parsley, savory, mace, onion powder, black pepper, and sage.

Taste is a personal thing, but if you're willing to experiment, you can find new ways to please your own palate. Marinades can be made with table wine, vinegar, and oil or unsalted salad dressings. The American Heart Association suggests lemon juice, vinegar, Tabasco sauce, or unsalted liquid smoke for adding flavor to meats, soups, and vegetables.

America was discovered because the world craved herbs

and spices—and a shorter route to the lands where they grew. If you're on a lower-salt diet, it's your turn to play Columbus. To help you explore these new tastes, here is a chart of what herbs and spices go best with which foods. Remember that dried herbs are stronger than fresh ones. If you're using fresh and a recipe calls for dried, use twice the amount. If you're using dried and the recipe calls for fresh, use half the amount.

TABLE 3. Flavor Adventures*

MEAT FISH POULTRY	*Beef:* Bay leaf, dry mustard powder, green pepper, marjoram, fresh mushrooms, nutmeg, onion, pepper, sage, thyme.
	Chicken: Green pepper, lemon juice, marjoram, fresh mushrooms, paprika, parsley, poultry seasoning, sage, thyme.
	Fish: Bay leaf, curry powder, dry mustard powder, green pepper, lemon juice, marjoram, fresh mushrooms, paprika.
	Lamb: Curry powder, garlic, mint, mint jelly, pineapple, rosemary.
	Pork: Apple, applesauce, garlic, onion, sage.
	Veal: Apricot, bay leaf, curry powder, ginger, marjoram, oregano.
VEGETABLES	*Asparagus:* Garlic, lemon juice, onion, vinegar.
	Corn: Green pepper, pimento, fresh tomato.
	Cucumbers: Chives, dill, garlic, vinegar.
	Green Beans: Dill, lemon juice, marjoram, nutmeg, pimento.
	Peas: Green pepper, mint, fresh mushrooms, onion, parsley.
	Potatoes: Green pepper, onion, pimento, saffron.
	Squash: Brown sugar, cinnamon, ginger, mace, nutmeg, onion.
	Tomatoes: Basil, marjoram, onion, oregano.
SOUP	*Soups:* A pinch of dry mustard powder in bean soup; allspice, a small amount of vinegar, or a dash of sugar in vegetable soup; peppercorns in skim-milk chowders; bay leaf and parsley in pea soup.

8. The Great Salt Debate

When the cause of a disease is a mystery, the cure is often a controversy. And that's what's happening here.

With high blood pressure, the most heated argument is over salt. Should you cut back on it or shouldn't you?

Traditionally, doctors have advised people with high blood pressure to go on a lower-salt diet. Most doctors continue to advise that. The American Medical Association, the American Heart Association, the American College of Physicians, and other respected groups all would agree with that. During his term as commissioner of the Food and Drug Administration, Arthur Hull Hayes, Jr., went even a step further. He championed the idea of making it "a general health goal for our nation" to reduce salt for everyone, regardless of their blood pressure.

Yet new voices are being heard from. There's a challenge now to the accepted idea that salt is necessarily bad for everyone. Among the leaders of this new school of thought are Dr. John H. Laragh, director of the Hypertension Center at The New York Hospital–Cornell Medical Center in New York, and Dr. David A. McCarron, director of the hypertension program at Oregon Health Sciences University.

Dr. Laragh is a man who likes to talk about "the great virtues of salt." He suggests that it's all right for some people with high blood pressure—but not all of them—to slip into the nearest delicatessen and order a corned beef on rye. It could even be okay to eat the sour pickle that comes with the sandwich.

"I am not against lowering salt for those who need it," explains Dr. Laragh. "I am only reacting to those who have overreacted and gone much too far with this."

These days, as he points out, antisalt is a popular medical opinion but not yet a proven fact. It is true that in some isolated cultures, such as a primitive tribe in the Solomon Islands in the Pacific, there is hardly any salt in the diet and hardly any hypertension. It is also true that in a high-salt civilization like our own, there's a high rate of hypertension. Yet it may not be good science to compare different cultures. Genetic differences, life-style differences, stress and climate differences, all sorts of other differences may help to account for the difference in hypertension.

"Within any given society," says Dr. Laragh, "there's no proof that less salt for everyone would mean longer life." In the famous Framingham, Massachusetts, study of heart disease, there was no difference in the amount of salt eaten by people who developed high blood pressure and people who didn't. In recent studies in Israel and in the United States, people with hypertension have lowered their pressure by losing weight but without changing the amount of salt they ate.

"Everybody with high blood pressure doesn't have the same disease," explains Dr. Laragh. According to his research and that of other medical scientists, the different forms of high blood pressure divide in this way:

- In about 30 percent of hypertension, salt is a major factor. These are the people who can lower their pressure by lowering the amount of salt they use and/or using a diuretic to eliminate the excess salt in their bodies.
- In another 30 percent, according to Dr. Laragh, the major factor is too much renin, a hormone manufactured by the kidneys. A low-salt diet won't help these people, Dr.

Laragh claims, and may harm them. This form of the disease is sometimes connected to a lack of calcium, and a low-salt diet may cut back on calcium-rich foods such as dairy products.

• In still another 30 percent, there's a combination problem with both renin and salt out of balance. Some of these people may be helped by a lower-salt diet; some may not.

• In the remaining 10 percent, the problem is physical. For some of these people, a new, simple, nonsurgical procedure, balloon dilation, can open up the blocked kidney arteries and so cure the disease.

A half-dozen years ago, hardly anyone believed in these subtypes of hypertension. Today, most doctors will admit that the different types do exist, but they don't always agree with Dr. Laragh's percentages. Nor do they seem to think that the different forms are very important. The medical consensus is to treat most high blood pressure by lowering salt. Renin still gets little attention, although Dr. Laragh reports that he's been able to partially or totally correct high blood pressure in seventy percent of his cases by giving a new drug, captopril, that works specifically against renin.

Who's right about salt? Each side finds it hard to come up with the proof that would convince the other side. The final answer may lie in the many and varied research studies that continue to be done on high blood pressure.

For today, though, there is a new test, the renin-sodium profile, that can reveal which type of hypertension is at work. Some doctors find the test accurate and helpful. Others claim that it doesn't always provide enough information, and so they don't want to put their patients to the expense of it.

Still, even at forty or fifty dollars, the test could be cheaper for some people than spending a great deal of time on the wrong drug or diet. Here and there, some doctors do feel that the test is especially helpful in spotting those people whose high blood pressure has a physical cause, such as a blockage in the kidney arteries.

Medical controversies such as this one tend to leave the patient bewildered and stranded somewhere in the middle of all the arguments. In this case, though, there's a way out. Some people may want to do their own bit of medical research.

If your doctor prescribes an antisalt drug or diet, agree to follow the prescription. Dr. Laragh suggests a week, but a month may sound more reasonable to your doctor. If your blood pressure comes down, you've pretty-well proven that salt was guilty in your case. If it doesn't come down, you may want to ask your doctor to do the new test, the renin-sodium profile, to find out more about what kind of hypertension is at work in your body.

9. New Ideas—and Answers

The more science knows, the more it knows that it needs to know. Yet it is becoming very clear that the food you eat—and the ways that your body deals with the elements of that food—can have a significant effect on your blood pressure.

The minerals in your food—ions such as calcium, magnesium, and potassium—are "the new frontier of blood-pressure research," according to Dr. Lawrence Resnick of The New York Hospital–Cornell Medical Center in New York City. You can't taste an ion or see it with the naked eye, but medical science is beginning to unravel the mysterious ways in which those ions work on blood pressure.

For some people, this could mean new and different dietary changes. Nobody, of course, should make such changes without consulting a physician.

The Calcium Connection

The evidence is small but dramatic—and growing. A "smoking-gun" link between calcium and high blood pressure was found by Dr. David McCarron, professor of medicine at Oregon Health Sciences University in Portland. He studied the dietary habits of a group of 90 adults, and he discovered that the 46 people who had high blood pressure ate significantly less calcium than the 44 others who had normal blood pressure.

There is other evidence that too little calcium can lead to too much blood pressure. Some of it is to be found in animal studies, some in surveys of human beings. At New York Hospital, Drs. Laragh and Resnick found that it depended on the patient's level of renin. For people who were low in renin, short-term calcium-loading—giving a patient vast amounts of extra calcium—brought about a significant lowering in blood pressure. For people who were higher in renin, it was magnesium-loading, rather than calcium, that lowered the blood pressure.

As Dr. Resnick explains, it's important to treat the individual, not the disease. "Just as salt isn't bad for everyone, calcium isn't good for everyone," he says. "The important thing is that we have the renin profile test, so we can tell who can be helped by what."

The way that calcium works is complicated and contradictory. It is involved in both the contraction and the relaxation of blood vessels. Some people have too much calcium in the cells of the walls of their blood vessels. That makes the vessels contract and raises the blood pressure.

Curiously, one cure for that is to *add* calcium to the diet. Doctors aren't sure why that works but, pragmatically, they have seen that it does. Adding calcium seems to adjust the way that the body metabolizes calcium, both intracellularly and extracellularly.

This effect of calcium is why some doctors worry about lowering salt for everyone. That would ban some of the high-salt foods—dairy products such as cheeses and yogurt—that also are high-calcium foods.

When calcium is the problem, there also are new drugs, calcium antagonists such as Verapamil, Nifedipine, and Diltiazem. These drugs act as gatekeepers, keeping the calcium from entering the walls of the blood vessels.

By happy chance, some of the older drugs also turn out to help with calcium. Thiazide diuretics are among the most commonly prescribed drugs for high blood pressure. They are given to flush out water and, along with it, excess salt.

Doctors now are finding that these drugs also work to improve the body's balance of calcium, thus lowering the blood pressure in two ways.

The Potassium Problem

Here again, the problem is not too much but too little of something. Potassium is a mineral that's essential to the body. It's needed to help keep the balance between the cells and the body fluids. It plays a role in the response of nerves to stimulation and in the contraction of muscles. It's important for the functioning of certain enzymes.

It's also linked to blood pressure. "Low potassium is not a cause of blood pressure, but it can exacerbate the condition," explains Dr. Michael Horan of the Division of Heart and Vascular Disease of the National Heart, Lung, and Blood Institute, one of the National Institutes of Health.

Low potassium may be there on its own, perhaps because of diet. Or it can be a side effect of some blood-pressure medications. As they flush out water and salt to lower the blood pressure, some diuretics also lower the body's level of potassium.

There is growing evidence that by adding potassium, some people can lower their blood pressure. Some doctors manage this by prescribing potassium in concentrated powder or pill form. Other doctors suggest that you eat potassium-rich foods.

If your doctor has advised that you increase your potassium, the following chart can help you to find the best foods for doing that. Your doctor will tell you how much additional potassium you need, but generally 2,000 milligrams is the amount that's often advised.

For people who've also been told to watch their sodium, the chart indicates the amount of sodium in a serving of each food. (Note that canned or processed foods often have sodium added, so check the labels.) For those who also are watching their weight, we've divided the list according to the number of calories in a serving of each food.

TABLE 4. Potassium and Sodium Content of Foods*

Very Good Sources 400 Milligrams Potassium or More per Serving	Milli-grams Sodium	*Good Sources* 200–400 Milligrams Potassium per Serving	Milli-grams Sodium	*Fair Sources* 100–200 Milligrams Potassium per Serving	Milli-grams Sodium
100 Calories or Less per Serving					
Banana, 1 medium	1	Artichoke, bud or globe	46	All-Bran, ¼ cup	121
Cantaloupe, 1 cup	19			Apple, medium	1
Grapefruit juice, 1 cup	1	Beets, cooked, ½ cup	73	Apricots, canned, 3 halves	1
		Beet greens, ½ cup	55	Apricots, dried, sulfured, 5 halves	6
Honeydew melon, 1 cup	20	Blackberries, 1 cup	1	Asparagus, cooked, ½ cup	1
Molasses, 2 tablespoons	3	Broccoli, cooked, ½ cup	8	Bean sprouts, ½ cup	3
				Blueberries, 1 cup	1
				Bran flakes, ¾ cup	156
Nectarine, 1 large	8	Brussels sprouts, fresh, ½ cup	8	Cabbage, cooked, ½ cup	15
				Carrots, cooked, ½ cup	25
				Cauliflower, cooked, ½ cup	6
Orange juice, 1 cup	2	Buttermilk (low fat), 1 cup	319	Celery, 3- to 5-inch stalks	63
Potato baked, 1 medium	4			Cherries, raw, 15 large	2
Potato, boiled, pared before cooking, 1 medium	2	Carrots, raw, 1 large	34	Cole slaw (made with salad dressing), ½ cup	75
		Collard greens, cooked, frozen, ½ cup	14	Corn, cooked, fresh, ½ cup	1
				Corn, fresh, 1 small ear	1

Fruit cocktail, ½ cup	12	Eggplant, cooked, ½ cup	1
Nonfat dry milk powder, ¼ cup	89	Figs, canned in syrup, 3 medium	2
Orange, 1 small	1	Grapefruit, canned, ½ cup	2
		Grapefruit, medium, ½	2
Peach, raw, 1 medium	1	Grapes, 15	3
Pear, raw, 1 medium	3	Green beans, cooked, ½ cup	3
Potato, mashed, ½ cup (milk and tablespoon fat added)	348	Green pepper, 1 medium	10
		Lettuce, 4 large leaves	1
		Mushrooms, raw, ½ cup	11
		Mustard greens, ½ cup	12
		Okra, cooked, 10 pods	2
Rutabaga, cooked, ½ cup	7	Peas, cooked, ½ cup	2
		Pineapple, canned, 1 slice	1
Skim milk, 1 cup	127	Plums, 3	1
Spinach, cooked, ½ cup	90	Radishes, 10 medium	15
		Summer squash, cooked, ½ cup	1
Strawberries, frozen, sliced, 1 cup	3	Tangerine, 1 large	2
		Turnip greens, frozen, ½ cup	14
Tomatoes, cooked, canned, ½ cup	157		
Tomato, raw	3		
Watermelon, 2 cups	4		
Winter squash, frozen, cooked, ½ cup	1		

TABLE 4. Potassium and Sodium Content of Foods* (continued)

Very Good Sources 400 Milligrams Potassium or More per Serving	Milligrams Sodium	*Good Sources* 200–400 Milligrams Potassium per Serving	Milligrams Sodium	*Fair Sources* 100–200 Milligrams Potassium per Serving	Milligrams Sodium
100–200 Calories per Serving					
Avocado, ½	5	Apple juice, 1 cup	2	Cherries, canned, ½ cup	2
Flounder, baked, 3 ounces	66	Beef, lean, cooked, 3 ounces	51	Pineapple juice, 1 cup	3
		Chicken, cooked, (light) 3 ounces	54	Walnuts, 14 halves or 1 ounce	1
Halibut, baked, 3 ounces	45	Chicken, cooked (dark), 3 ounces	72		
Prunes, 10 medium	9	Chickpeas or garbanzos, ½ cup	19		
Prune juice, ¾ cup	4	Lamb, lean, cooked, 3 ounces	53		
Soybeans, cooked, ½ cup	2	Lentils, cooked, ½ cup	19		
		Lima beans, green, ½ cup	1		
		Parsnips, cooked, ½ cup	6		

		Peaches, canned, 2 halves	4		
		Peanut butter, 2 table-spoons	97		
		Pork, lean, 3 ounces	51		
		Raisins, natural-unbleached, ⅓ cup or 1½-ounce pkg.	12		
		Red beans, cooked, ½ cup	10		
		Salmon, pink, canned, 3 ounces	375		
		Split peas, cooked, ½ cup	14		
		Sunflower seeds, hulled, ¼ cup	11		
		Sweet potato, canned, ½ cup	52		
		Tuna fish, ½ cup	500		
		Turkey, light, 3 ounces	69		
		Turkey, dark, 3 ounces	75		
		Veal, 3 ounces	51		
		White beans, cooked, ½ cup	7		
200 Calories or More per Serving					
Dates, 10 medium	1	Peanuts, shelled, ¼ cup	2		
Figs, dried, 5 medium	10				

10. Exercise and Blood Pressure

Whatever else your doctor may have told you to do about your blood pressure, did he or she also add one final admonition? Did the doctor say, ". . . and get some exercise"?

That mild statement represents a revolution in medical thinking. At one time, doctors thought that physical exercise was dangerous for people with hypertension or coronary heart disease. These people were told to shun all exertion. "Take it easy," the doctor used to say. "Don't run. Don't climb any stairs."

Today, that's all changed. Now, exercise is often part of the prescription. Can physical exercise really bring down your diastolic? Can you literally run away from your blood pressure?

When you exercise, a great many things happen in your body. There is a small but growing literature of research that suggests that some of these things have a direct effect on your blood pressure. There is massive, convincing evidence that other things have indirect benefits. Exercise has a positive effect on your heart, on your weight, and on your state of mind, and these improvements can be helpful, even lifesaving, to someone with high blood pressure.

According to Dr. Thomas G. Pickering, the people most likely to benefit from physical exercise are those with mild or borderline hypertension. As we've told you, that's the zone, the gray area, where the diastolic is 90 to 104, where most hypertensives find themselves.

How much exercise? For how long? How strenuous? The answers depend on your general physical condition. Usually, it's wise to begin slowly and build up from there. Always, it's very important to consult with a physician before starting any program of exercise.

It takes motivation to start a program and stay with it. A quick look at some of the proof of what exercise can do for you may be an incentive to get up, get out, get going.

The Direct Link

About ten years ago, worried about his own high blood pressure, Dr. Robert Cade began to jog every afternoon. As his own diastolic fell back down to normal, the physician wondered if he could cure other people in the same way.

A professor of medicine at the University of Florida at Gainesville, Dr. Cade studied the relationship between high blood pressure and exercise. In the laboratory, he worked with 370 hypertensive volunteers, measuring their pressure before and after fast-paced rides on a stationary bicycle. "About ninety-six percent of the patients showed a significant drop in blood pressure after three months of exercise," he reports. The improvements were dramatic, ranging from 10 to 50 downward points.

Other studies have also shown significant, though more modest, changes. It's not clear whether Dr. Cade's patients also lost weight, a factor that could have contributed to their lower pressure. In at least one other study, though, there were important changes in blood pressure without any changes in weight.

Generally, people who are physically fit tend to have lower blood pressure than people who lead sedentary lives. One difference between those who exercise and those who don't is in the levels of blood viscosity. If the blood is thick and syrupy—in medical language, viscous—that increases the resistance or pressure of its flow through the blood vessels. Recently, in his work at the Hypertension Center at New York Hospital, Dr. Pickering has observed that people with high blood pressure tend to have high levels of blood viscosity. People who exercise have lower levels than those who don't exercise, and so it looks as if exercise may help to lower the blood pressure by lowering the blood viscosity.

Exercise and Your Heart

One of the urgent reasons for wanting to lower your blood pressure is the worry over what a high pressure can mean to your heart. High blood pressure can lead to a heart attack, but exercise can lead away from it. In study after study, it's been shown that exercise reduces the risk of cardiovascular problems.

When you first begin to exercise vigorously, your heart will seem to pound. The rate at which it is beating goes way up. After a while, as you exercise regularly, the heart muscles become stronger and the heart rate doesn't go up as much. The beat becomes steadier and slower, both when you're exercising and when you're performing your normal daily tasks. That's especially beneficial for people whose blood-pressure problems include a narrowing of the arteries.

Exercise has another boon for your heart. By changing your metabolism, it seems to have an effect on the body's cholesterol, increasing the good lipids in the cholesterol as opposed to the bad, life-threatening ones.

Exercise and Your Diet

Lowering your weight can help to lower your blood pressure. In itself, exercise can help you to take off some pounds. In addition, it helps whatever diet you're on to work better.

People used to worry, for example, that exercise would stimulate their appetites and lead them to eat more. We now know that exercise works in exactly the opposite way. It's an appetite suppressant, and sometimes can stave off that hungry feeling for hours.

Exercise also seems to step up the body's idling speed. For as long as fifteen hours after you've exercised vigorously, according to some research, your body will continue to burn calories at a higher rate than if you hadn't exercised. If you exercise once in the morning and then again in the evening, you can be burning up your calories at that higher rate around the clock. In other words, you may be losing weight even while you sleep.

Timing is important. Researchers at Cornell University have found that it's best to exercise within two or three hours after eating a meal. Doing the same amount of exercise, your body burns up more calories than if you were exercising on an empty stomach.

With exercise, you lose body fat—the tissue that burns calories slowly—and build up muscle—the tissue that burns calories more quickly. In that way, it becomes possible to lose more weight with the same number of calories.

Exercise and Feeling Good

People with high blood pressure need to learn to deal better with the daily stresses and strains that can send their pressure soaring. Exercise can help here, too.

Exercise triggers the release of the body's own natural mood-improver, a calming chemical called beta-endorphin. That's what causes the "runner's high" that you may have heard about. It's there with any vigorous exercise, the body's way of making the mind feel good.

In the Perrier Survey of Fitness in America, a nationwide survey conducted by the Louis Harris polling organization, people who exercise regularly were more likely to think of themselves as relaxed, optimistic, not subject to depression, energetic, and disciplined. People who don't exercise were much less likely to describe themselves in those positive ways. It could be the endorphins released by exercise that make people feel so self-affirming. Or it could simply be that feeling good about your body is a giant step toward feeling good about your total self.

Exercise seems to lead people to choose a different lifestyle. When doctors tour the intensive-care unit, they often recognize the person who's lying there. All too often, he's that familiar high-risk person—the overweight, hypertensive, high-cholesterol, sedentary, type-A smoker. People who exercise seem more likely to avoid that fatal list of risk factors. Vigorous exercise seems to bring about changes in the compulsive, striving type-A behavior pattern. In the Perrier study, people who exercised smoked less and paid more attention to the kinds of food they ate than did other people.

What Kind of Exercise?

Even mild exercise can change your metabolism. To get the full cardiovascular effect and the calorie-burning effect, though, it takes aerobic exercise. That's the kind of exercise that sets your heart to pounding and your blood to racing, the kind of exercise that pushes many different sets of muscles to continuous movement.

Jogging may be the first aerobic exercise that comes to mind. It's an ideal one, but many doctors now feel that brisk walking can be just as effective for some people. Other good choices include cross-country skiing, jumping rope, bicycle riding (on the road or on a stationary cycle), swimming, aerobic dancing or calisthenics, roller skating, even disco dancing.

The exercise you enjoy is the one you're most apt to stick to, and so that's the basis on which to choose your aerobic. Some people find that it's easier to stay with jogging or brisk walking if they do it with a companion. Others find that a dance or exercise class—with the need to be at a specific place at a specific time—provides the discipline they need. Still others find that exercise is more interesting if they alternate between two or three different forms of aerobics.

The ideal is to exercise every day. If you can't fit that into your schedule, then three times a week, twenty minutes at a time, is the minimum if you want to get the genuine benefits of aerobic exercise.

The benefits begin as soon as your program of exercise begins. In itself, it may take three or four months for exercise alone to bring about a measurable change in your blood pressure. Along with other things you're doing—such as dieting or learning to deal better with stress—it can be an important help in lowering your pressure in a matter of weeks.

An Exercise Bonus

If you need an extra incentive to start exercising, consider this: People who exercise regularly may be better decision makers. In a recent study at Purdue University, that was the finding of Professor Gavriel Salvendy, chair of Purdue's Interdisciplinary Graduate Program in Human Factors and a professor in the School of Industrial Engineering. His research showed that people involved in a regular fitness program made sixty percent fewer errors in forming strategies to arrive at complex decisions.

So make a good decision for yourself—and start exercising.

11. Relax: The Take-It-Easy Way to Health

When our ancestor the caveman was faced with a wild tiger, his heart began to race, his breathing came faster, his blood pressure soared. Oxygen, adrenaline, and other substances were being pumped to the muscles, girding them to do what was necessary for survival—either fight the tiger or run from it.

That's the fight-or-flight response, an automatic, coordinated series of reactions that the human body evolved to deal with emergencies.

Today, few of us are confronted by wild beasts, but daily life can be a parade of paper tigers. An ambulance goes by, sirens screaming. Someone cuts in front of you in a line of traffic. You argue with someone you love. The phone rings. You're rushing to get to work on time. You're called in to your boss's office. You have a report to deliver, a test to take, a party to attend.

You can't fight these events, at least not physically. Nor can you flee from them. Yet your body still reacts with the fight-or-flight response. You may not be aware of it, but your heart is pounding, your blood is rushing, your pressure is climbing.

The emergency response that saved the caveman's life can be dangerous to his descendants. It can have harmful effects, straining your system. If it takes place too often, it can raise the blood pressure—and keep it raised. If the blood pressure is high to begin with, that soaring blood pressure can be life threatening.

There is no escape from the rush, the clamor, the jingle and jangle of modern life. There is no way to avoid the fight-or-flight response, but there is a way to tame it. Each of us has within us the ability to set off a series of reactions that are just the opposite of the emergency response.

A Positive Answer

The counterresponse is called the relaxation response. Developed by Dr. Herbert Benson of the Harvard Medical School, this is a way to decrease and counteract the negative effects of the emergency response. It's a way of replacing those health-threatening effects with health-enhancing ones.

In research with people who have high blood pressure, Dr. Benson taught the relaxation response to men and women and then monitored their pressure. After they'd been using the relaxation response for a few weeks, he found that, on the average, people had lowered their systolic from 146 to 137 and brought their diastolic down from 93.5 to 88.9. That's a significant change, large enough to bring people from borderline hypertension to normal.

Most important of all, that lower blood pressure was there at times of the day when people were not practicing the relaxation response. In other words, the relaxation brought the pressure down—and then kept it down.

The effects of the emergency response are set in motion by a rush of bodily hormones. Some of the drugs that are used to control high blood pressure work by blocking the response of those hormones. The relaxation response seems to work in the same way, just like a drug, but without side effects. And just as a drug continues to work after you've swallowed it, so the relaxation response continues to work after you've elicited it. With it, you can lower your blood pressure—and keep it low.

That's a large promise, but it can be kept.

The relaxation response sounds simple. And, as you'll see, it is.

How to Get the Relaxation Response

There are five easy-to-follow steps to bringing about the relaxation response.

Step One: Find a quiet area and a comfortable chair. Sit down, taking any position that feels easy and natural to you.

Step Two: Close your eyes.

Step Three: Think to yourself or speak aloud—whichever you prefer—a repetitive word, sound, or phrase. Try not to be conscious of any other words, sounds, or thoughts. Some people like to repeat a word or phrase that's meaningful to them, perhaps a prayer. Others choose a word that's calming and neutral, like "one."

Step Four: Breathe through your nose and try to keep your breathing regular and rhythmical. Each time you breathe out, repeat your word or sound. If any other words or thoughts come into your mind, push them away, perhaps just by telling them "Go away" or "Not now."

Step Five: Continue this for fifteen or twenty minutes. When that period of time is up, stay seated—first with your eyes closed, then with eyes opened—for a few minutes before picking up the threads of your life.

To get the full benefit, this needs to be done twice a day, for fifteen or twenty minutes each time. To make it a habit, a regular part of your daily life, try to choose the same times each day for this relaxing exercise. Some people like to schedule it once in the morning and then again in the evening. At work, other people find their efficiency goes up if they use their coffee break for a "relaxation break." If you're a commuter, this could be a good use of your time on the bus or train.

Don't set an alarm clock to signal when the relaxation time is up. That's too nerve jangling. If you find yourself wondering how much time has passed, though, it's all right to open your eyes and look briefly at your watch.

If you're especially tense, you may want to add an extra step, progressive relaxation, just after the regular Step Two. To do this, relax your muscles, beginning with your toes and working up to your neck and head. Do this progressively, one set of muscles at a time. First tense your toes, then relax them. Now the muscles in the arch of your foot. Next the calf muscles. The thighs. And so on. Think of each muscle or set of muscles separately, relax them, and then continue, until your entire body feels free of tension.

Feeling Better

During his fifteen years of research on relaxation and its effect on the heart and the blood pressure, Dr. Benson has worked with large numbers of people. As he says, "The great majority of people report feelings of relaxation and freedom from anxiety during the elicitation of the relaxation response and during the rest of the day, as well."

Your own feelings are a good measurement, but not a scientific one. The relaxation response is a good idea for anybody, regardless of blood pressure. It is a risk-free tonic for mind and body. Still, if you're using it in order to try to lower your blood pressure, you should talk to your doctor about it first.

The relaxation response brings about actual physiological changes, and those have been measured in the controlled conditions of the laboratory. Without that scientific monitoring, the average person can't know for certain whether the meditation is really eliciting the response and whether those physiological changes—such as a lower blood pressure—actually are taking place.

That's why it's important to do this in partnership with your doctor. Then you and the doctor can arrange to check your blood pressure at regular intervals, to measure the effect of the relaxation response. For some people, especially those in the mild or borderline zones, the relaxation response may be able to bring pressure down to normal without any medication. For others, especially those whose pressure is higher, the relaxation response may be something to add to your diet or to the pills that are now being taken. Used along with medication, the relaxation response acts to enhance the way the drug works, and this can lead eventually to fewer drugs or lower dosages.

With drugs or without them, depending on the advice of your doctor, the relaxation response is not a "cure." It must continue to be used in order to continue to work, lowering and controlling your blood pressure. It begins to work quickly, though. If you're using it properly, you should see changes in your blood pressure in thirty days.

The Nonbelievers

When you talk to your doctor about the relaxation response, you may be met with skepticism. Not all physicians are convinced that it works.

There are a number of studies, apart from those Dr. Benson has done, that show that it can lower blood pressure and keep it down. In some other studies, though, blood pressure went down very little or not at all. In some, if the pressure went down, it didn't stay down for very long after the relaxation.

There is an odd truth about research on human beings. Somehow, researchers tend to get the results they expect to get. Through tone of voice, looks, gestures, body posture, the researcher sends a message to the subject. There's an unspoken dialogue between them. Often, that leads to the result—pro or con—that the researcher may have wanted or expected all along.

Like the researcher, each person also gets the result he or she wants. Anything—medication or meditation—works better if you believe in it. Any therapy is more successful if the patient has faith that it will work. That's why some people are "cured" of major diseases by placebos or sugar pills.

When you believe in something, your brain sends a positive message to the body, ordering up positive physiological and biochemical changes. Paul J. Rosch, M.D., president of the American Institute of Stress, explains it this way:

"What happens when you undergo any therapy—whether it's chemotherapy at Sloan-Kettering, or faith healing, or visualizing that your white cells are attacking a tumor—is that you say to yourself, 'Hey, look, I'm taking control of this thing.' Somehow the brain translates that message so that the immune system understands it and acts on it."

The relaxation response can help to send that positive message—if you believe in it.

How It Works

Back in junior high school, the science teacher may have told you about the two nervous systems. There was the voluntary nervous system for the things we can control. Through this system, we will our feet to walk, our arms to reach out, our mouths to speak. And there was the involuntary, or autonomic, nervous system, for the things we don't have control over, such inner processes as heart rate, digestion—and blood pressure.

Today, doctors speak more and more of a single nervous system, everything working together, interdependent, the mind affected by the body, the body touched by the mind. Now we're finding that the mind can have an effect on those hidden processes of the body. Relaxation is one of the ways that we can control what once seemed uncontrollable.

For a number of years now, a few people have been learning to control their blood pressure through a complicated process known as biofeedback. Hooked up to a monitor, they learn how it feels when the machine beeps that their pressure is high and how it feels when the signal says it's normal. With time, they learn to bring about the right signal and then to do it without the machine. Some people become so adept that they can change the flow of blood in one ear but not the other.

Biofeedback is difficult and expensive, and many people cannot learn to do it. These days, a growing number of doctors are working on simpler, easy-to-learn techniques that achieve the same end, lowering the pressure.

While you're relaxing or meditating, for example, a number of physical changes take place. The rate of breathing slows down, dropping by about two breaths per minute in most people. Those people who have meditated for many years, though, sometimes seem to have stopped breathing.

In the laboratory, they've been measured as low as zero to one breath a minute for three to four minutes on end.

During the relaxation response, the amount of oxygen the body uses decreases. The heart rate slows down. Muscle tension ebbs. And the blood pressure goes down.

There's a change, too, in the pattern of brain waves. There is an increase in the amount of alpha waves, the ones associated with calm and peaceful feelings.

Another change is a precipitous drop in arterial blood lactate, "to some of the lowest levels ever recorded in humans," according to Dr. Benson. High levels of lactate are connected with states of anxiety and disquiet. Low levels are associated with peace and tranquility.

What's even more important—and more remarkable—is that these changes don't end when the meditation ends. When Dr. Benson compared people who didn't meditate with those who did, he found physiologic differences. The series of bodily changes that begin with relaxation and then continue are changes that revolve around a decrease in the body's response to norepinephrine, the excitement hormone that causes the heart to speed up and the blood pressure to rise. Both groups of people—those who practiced the relaxation response and those who didn't—were still producing that hormone. The difference was that, hours later, those who practiced the relaxation response were no longer reacting to the hormone in the same agitated way. "Even when you're not eliciting the relaxation response," explains Dr. Benson, "it leads to physiologic changes within the body that carry over for prolonged periods of time, acting essentially as many drugs do."

For a number of years now, they've been observing this at the Beth Israel Hospital in Boston and at other research centers. According to these studies, truly relaxing the mind and the body mimics the effect that some blood-pressure pills would have. The system stays calm, less vulnerable to stress. The blood pressure stays lower for long after you've stopped meditating and have returned to the tensions and demands of ordinary life.

Tested by Time

The relaxation response is an old and time-honored idea in a new and scientific form. At first thought, meditation may seem like something that Americans "discovered" in the 1960's, when there was an explosion of interest in Oriental religions, when Zen and Yoga became the rage, when maharishis seemed to be everywhere.

East and West, though, this is something people everywhere have been doing for thousands of years. Meditation is part of some Oriental religions but it is in the mainstream of Western religions as well.

Tracing its history in religious and secular writings, Dr. Benson has found countless references that sound very much like the relaxation response. Again and again, in almost every human culture, there's a description of the same steps to relaxation. People may not have understood the medical implications, but they did know that it made them feel better, calmer, more in tune with the world around them, and, for some, closer to God.

The search through the past took Dr. Benson all the way back to the seventh century B.C. At that time, in the Upanishads, the Hindu scriptures, it was written that to achieve a union with God, you should sit quietly, pay attention to your breathing, and, each time you exhale, repeat silently a word of praise from the scripture. If other thoughts came to mind, the seeker was instructed to passively disregard them and return to the repetition.

Another ancient example was found within Judaism, going back to the time of the Second Temple, in a tradition called merkabolism. Squatting in the fetal position, people would rock from heel to toe and, on each out-breath, repeat over and over the name of the magic seal.

In Christianity, there are prayers that date from the time of Jesus Christ. Those prayers were passed on by word of mouth through the monasteries, then codified in the fourteenth century at Mount Athos in Greece. There, to this day, they are part of life in the Byzantine monasteries. The instructions were twice daily to sit quietly by yourself, pay attention to your breathing, and, each time you breathe out, recite the prayer "Lord Jesus Christ, have mercy." If other thoughts came to mind, the believer was told to ignore them and go back to the repetition of the prayer. In modern Catholicism and also in modern Episcopalianism, this survives as "the Jesus prayer," or the prayer of the heart. The Greek Orthodox tradition has similar prayers.

In northern Europe, during the Middle Ages when the Jewish cabalistic tradition was evolving, a rabbi wrote, "To achieve the state, sit quietly, pay attention to your breathing, and on each out-breath, repeat the components that make up God's name, *Adonai.*"

There are similar traditions in Zen Buddhism, Tibetan Buddhism, Shintoism, Taoism. The steps are always the same; only the words are different.

Outside the religious tradition, in New England of the 1800's, it was part of the Transcendental movement led by Ralph Waldo Emerson. In England, it was practiced by the poet Alfred Lord Tennyson, a man with a healthy ego. As the story goes, the word that he chose to repeat was his own name, saying it over and over again: Tennyson, Tennyson, Tennyson.

Good Stress—and Bad

Stress is a constant part of life, but not all of it is harmful. "A certain amount of stress is needed to tune up for action and keep you on your toes," wrote the late Hans Selye, the doctor and philosopher who is considered the father of stress research. He made the distinction between "distress," as he called the negative form of stress, and "eustress" (from the Greek prefix for "good," as in "euphoria"), as he called the positive form.

Without excitement, challenges, changes, stimulation—all of which can involve a degree of stress—life would be boring and monotonous. Boredom, listlessness, a sense that life has no purpose—these feelings can create their own forms of stress and take their own physical and mental toll. To avoid that, many of us go out looking for sources of stress. We seek challenges we can respond to on the ski slope or the golf course, at the card table or on the freeway.

"Each person has his or her own tolerance for stress," explains Dr. Leon J. Warshaw, a professor of environmental medicine at New York University. There's an optimal zone above which you feel too much stress and below which you can feel the stress of deprivation.

So the relaxation response is not meant to smooth out all of life's hills and valleys, just make the journey safer. It is not meant to stop you from revving up on the tennis court or at important meetings. It's not designed to stifle the pleasant flutter of excitement when you're making a speech or giving a party. It is meant to give you some control over how you respond, which is a way of giving you some control over your blood pressure. It can keep you from overreacting, mind and body, to the bustle, the clamor, the rush, the noise, the tensions and demands of daily life.

Stress is also the way we respond when we're called on to make a change in our daily life. It happens whether the change is for the good or for the bad. Whenever we are required to adjust our behavior to a new set of circumstances, the hormones begin to rage. Different life events cause different amounts of stress, and it's helpful to know what those are.

Drs. Thomas Holmes and Richard Rahe, both psychiatrists at the University of Washington Medical School, worked out a scale of life events. They interviewed hundreds of men and women of different ages, backgrounds, economic and social classes, asking about the adjustment to these events. Then they ranked the events according to the amount of stress each involved.

Which of these is happening in your life now? Which is yet another urgent reason to do something about your blood pressure?

THE SCALE OF LIFE EVENTS

Event	*Scale of stress*
Death of spouse	100
Divorce	73
Marital separation	65
Jail term	63
Death of close family member	63
Personal injury or illness	53

THE SCALE OF LIFE EVENTS

Event	*Scale of stress*
Marriage	50
Fired at work	47
Marital reconciliation	45
Retirement	45
Change in health of family member	44
Pregnancy	40
Sex difficulties	39
Gain of new family member	39
Business readjustment	39
Change in financial state	38
Death of close friend	37
Change to different line of work	36
Change in number of arguments with spouse	35
Mortgage over $10,000	31
Foreclosure of mortgage or loan	30
Change in responsibilities at work	29
Son or daughter leaving home	29
Trouble with in-laws	29
Outstanding personal achievement	28
Wife begins or stops work	26
Begin or end of school	26
Change in living conditions	25
Revision of personal habits	24
Trouble with boss	23
Change in work hours or conditions	20
Change in residence	20
Change in schools	20
Change in recreation	19
Change in church activities	19
Change in social activities	18
Mortgage or loan less than $10,000	17
Change in sleeping habits	16
Change in number of family get-togethers	15
Change in eating habits	15
Vacation	13
Christmas	12
Minor violations of the law	11

The Health Bonuses of Relaxation

When you're unable to cope with stress, your body rebels. Doctors have long known about the link between psychological or emotional stress and physical disease. Now, from Mt. Sinai Medical Center in New York and the University of Colorado, there's new evidence on how this works. According to the recent research, when stress is too great or lasts too long, it may weaken the body's immune system. That's the system that is responsible for fighting off disease. When it is weakened, people are more likely to develop cancer and other serious diseases.

No one has yet proved that if you learn to deal better with stress, you'll be less likely to get cancer. Yet there are a number of clinical studies that demonstrate the medical benefits and bonuses of the relaxation response.

With the relaxation response, Dr. Benson has been able to cure all sorts of pain and tension headaches. Working with migraine sufferers, he's found that about half of them are helped by this. More chronic pain, such as low back pain, can be significantly eased. Cardiac arrhythmias can be significantly decreased.

Do you have any of these problems? The relaxation response may help to ease them—a bonus to the other good-health benefits of improving your emotional state, protecting your heart, and lowering your blood pressure.

12. Talking Your Way Down

"I *want to lower my blood pressure."*

If you were to read that sentence out loud—even all alone in a room—your blood pressure would go up. If you read it aloud to someone else, it would go up still higher.

Suppose, instead of reading, you are talking to that other person. If you say something neutral, perhaps simply telling your name and address, that's enough to raise your blood pressure. If you are saying something that carries more emotion and more meaning—talking about your job, about your marriage partner, about politics—the increase would be higher yet.

These rises in blood pressure are natural and normal. They take place in everyone, young or old, male or female, with normal blood pressure or high blood pressure.

The amount of the increase when you're talking, though, depends on what your blood pressure is to begin with. The increase is greatest for those who can least afford it. For people with normal blood pressure, talking can raise it 10 or 20 points, depending on the situation. For people with high blood pressure, the rise can be as high as 50 points.

The link between communication and blood pressure is an important one. Talking is, after all, something we do all day long—at home and at work, on the phone and in the elevator, at the store and over the dinner table. Whether you're questioning a child about his report card or saying something as simple as "Please pass the salt," there's an effect on your blood pressure.

Doctors have only recently come to understand that effect. With this new understanding, they are developing new ideas about communication and new ways to control and lower your blood pressure.

The Vocabulary of Blood Pressure

The computer has come to the blood-pressure laboratory, and that's what makes it possible now to see the minute-by-minute changes that take place in everybody. With a microcomputer and an automated blood-pressure-cuff system, a person's blood pressure and heart rate now can be measured continuously. Every sixty seconds, the results are flashed onto a screen.

In this way, thousands of people have been studied in recent years by a team of doctors, nurses, and researchers, a team headed by James Lynch, Ph.D., professor of psychiatry and director of the Psychophysiological Clinic at the University of Maryland School of Medicine in Baltimore. They are finding that the changes in blood pressure are more dramatic in men, while the changes in heart rate are more marked in women. Both changes, though, are a challenge to health.

"Your pressure goes up within half a minute of your starting to speak," reports Dr. Lynch. The more emotional or stressful the topic, the steeper the rise. If it's something you're angry about, or if it's a secret you've decided to tell at last, both the systolic and the diastolic will soar.

The person you're talking to also makes a difference. If you're married, your blood pressure goes up less when you talk to someone of the opposite sex than if you're single. It's easier on the blood pressure for a boss to talk to a subordinate than vice versa.

If blood pressure zips up when you speak, it comes down just as quickly when you listen to the other person in the conversation. If, that is, you are really listening. In the laboratory, patients listen carefully to the doctor or nurse who is telling them what they want to know about their blood pressure. In everyday life, many of us don't listen well. We may be thinking "how silly" or "how boring" or "how wrong" the other person is. We may be planning how we're going to answer when it's our turn again. We may be getting ready to interrupt. If that's what's happening, then the pressure that went up as we were talking does not go down as fast or as far as when we're really listening.

Silence Isn't the Answer

People with high blood pressure tend to be poor communicators, according to Dr. Lynch. Their pressure goes up higher and stays up longer. That's a high cost to the cardiovascular system.

The answer is not to avoid communication. Alienation and loneliness take their own toll on health and well-being. Isolation can make you ill.

If you live like a hermit, apart, withdrawn, seldom talking to anyone, then any conversation that you do have can be a serious stress. "When you do have to talk to someone," explains Dr. Lynch, "you really overshoot your pressure."

Blood pressure goes up more in conversations with strangers, less in talking to good friends, husbands, wives, and lovers. In bereavement, when someone loses a beloved husband or wife, they've also lost the person they feel most comfortable with, the one that it's easiest to speak to. Something precious to health is gone, and the survivor is left to speak to a world of strangers.

For all of us, intimacy is important. The human being is a social animal. "The last time we did a survey in our hospital," notes Dr. Lynch, "fifty-two percent of the patients in the coronary care unit had been living alone when they were admitted."

We are communicating creatures, though some of us need to learn to do that better.

A New, Better Way of Talking

The better you can control any kind of stress, the better you can control your blood pressure. The more you ease your daily tensions, the more your pressure will ebb down to normal. If, on the other hand, your pressure is spurting too high too often as you relate and talk with other people, you can measure the cost in a higher blood pressure and a greater strain on your system.

The idea of lowering your blood pressure by improving your speech habits is a new one. Here and there, though, Dr. Lynch and other pioneers have been working with people with hypertension, trying to teach them to communicate better.

The results are remarkable and encouraging. Some of the patients at Dr. Lynch's Psychophysiological Clinic have been able to give up their blood-pressure pills, in consultation with their doctors. Others use the new techniques to make their medications work better, more effectively. Still others, people with normal pressure but a risk factor or two for higher pressure, are finding it good, preventive medicine.

Here, then, is a guide to better speech—and better health.

- *Slow down.* Dr. Lynch has found that people with high blood pressure tend to speak more rapidly than other people. That excitable tempo is part of what's bad for the blood pressure. Listen to yourself, and then try to moderate the tempo of words.

- *Put the commas in.* One way to improve the pattern of your speech is to think of the spoken word like the written word. In writing, the punctuation marks are signs that you're supposed to pause. In speaking, try to imagine those commas and semicolons and periods. Use them as pauses, as moments to come up for air. A few pauses or deep breaths between phrases, according to Dr. Lynch, can make a measurable difference in how high your pressure goes during speech. You may also find that it helps other people follow your meaning better than before.

• *Breathe slower.* As they talk quicker, hypertensives also tend to breathe quicker. Try to be aware of your breathing during conversations, and take deeper and more regular breaths.

• *Be aware of the people who make you tense.* Blood pressure goes up higher if you're talking to someone whose status is higher than yours. Your boss, for example. It's not practical to avoid those conversations, but it's helpful to be aware that this is a moment when you feel tense. Take a deep breath before you start to speak. Stay aware, so that your speech and breathing don't become too rapid.

• *Be aware of the subjects that make you tense.* Something that worries you, upsets you, or makes you feel resentful can push up your pressure. Try to know yourself better. What's bothering you? Is there something you can do or say to change that?

• *Be aware of situations that make you tense.* Is the telephone your bugaboo? Do you jump when it rings? Feel tense when you're dialing out? Some people find it helpful to paste a small blue circle on the phone dial. It's a reminder that this is something that makes them tense, a signal to take a deep breath first. Other people put those circles on the desk calendar, next to a meeting or appointment they feel nervous about. One of my neighbors has the circle on the inside door of the cabinet where she keeps the good china she uses when she's entertaining; it's her signal to relax and enjoy her own party.

• *Learn to listen better.* Try to pay attention to what the other person is saying. Try not to be critical or judgmental. Don't interrupt. Don't think about how you're going to answer. If you listen well, you're giving your blood pressure a chance to subside back to normal. You may also find that other people will enjoy talking to you more. If you think about the people who are described as good conversationalists, it's possible that they are good talkers; it's certain that they are good listeners.

- *Learn to relax.* Practice the relaxation response that's described in Chapter 11, or any other form of relaxation or meditation that you feel comfortable with. "Anything that lowers your overall pressure also lowers the amount it will go up when you speak," explains Dr. Lynch.

- *Stick with it for at least thirty days.* Changing the way you speak is easier said than done—but it can be done. With practice, you can slow your speech, slow your breathing, slow the rise in your pressure in thirty days.

13. Your Dialogue With the World

Think of a typical day. The people you meet. The sights you see. The noises you hear. Your feelings about all of that.

In countless and complex ways, each of us interacts with the people and the things around us. We respond to our environment. Aaron H. Katcher, M.D., professor of psychiatry at the University of Pennsylvania School of Medicine in Philadelphia, sums it up in a single word:

"Dialogue."

It's a way of saying that there's a constant exchange between us and the world around us. The ways we act, react, and interact can affect our health—for good or ill. They can add to our well-being or they can lead to such negative effects as migraine headaches, ulcers, irritable bowel syndrome—or high blood pressure.

Until recently, it was difficult to measure and demonstrate the effects of our dialogue. Now, with the same automated blood-pressure system as Dr. Lynch has been using, Dr. Katcher and others have been demonstrating that mind-and-body link.

For Dr. Katcher, the underlying cause of psychosomatic

disease may be in a person's dialogue. The cure may lie in changing that dialogue.

The Unspoken Dialogue

Other people are the major influence in anyone's life. Yet as Dr. Katcher points out, the dialogue we have with them is not always spoken out loud. A large part of it is silent. Each of us makes assumptions about the people around us, and then acts accordingly.

Take, for example, the dialogue at work. Why do two people who do the same job react so differently? Why does one feel relaxed and the other feel under great pressure?

"Different people make different assumptions," explains Dr. Katcher. Some people think that they can never do enough. They feel that they have to run as fast as they can, just to stay in the same place. They believe they have to do more and run faster, if they're going to get ahead. They expect that they'll never be able to do enough to satisfy the boss.

Other people have different expectations. They decide that the boss is a reasonable person. They assume that if they do their best, that's all anyone can ask. They, too, want to succeed, but they make assumptions that help them relax as they're doing it.

For almost everyone, blood pressure is higher at work than at home. The tenser you are about your job, though, the higher it will go. As Dr. Katcher explains, "A good deal depends not only on what the people around you actually do, but on what you *think* they're going to do."

What do you think your boss is thinking? What do you assume the people around you are feeling? Are you being reasonable? Does it match what, in fact, they actually do think and feel? For some people, a change in those assumptions could be the beginning of a change in blood pressure.

The Nonhuman Dialogue

We react to people, and our blood pressure goes up or down. We react to things, and the same process goes on.

We have a dialogue with sights and sounds. The jangle of a telephone. The wail of an ambulance. The stench that comes from a nearby factory. The garbage waiting to be picked up. The traffic jam on the thruway.

We can react to those stresses. Or we can respond to the pleasures around us. The tree that grows, even in Brooklyn. The white clouds scudding across a blue sky. The sound of a brook. The falling of snow.

"We can improve our dialogue and our blood pressure," advises Dr. Katcher, "by choosing what to concentrate on."

In an experiment, he asked people just to look at a tank full of tropical fish. He gave them no other instructions. After a few minutes, he checked their blood pressure. Among those people with normal blood pressure, it had fallen 10 to 12 points. Among those who had high blood pressure, it had dropped 18 to 20 points.

Relaxation—for People Who Can't Relax

As part of this therapy for people with hypertension, Dr. Katcher often recommends the relaxation response, developed by Dr. Herbert Benson and described in Chapter 11. Yet there are some people for whom that just doesn't work. They say they can't sit still for fifteen or twenty minutes. They're too impatient for a formal system of relaxation. Or they don't believe in it. Or they feel foolish sitting down and closing their eyes.

"I'm one of those people," admits Dr. Katcher. "I cannot continue with formal meditation." Yet for him, and for people like him, there's another, even simpler answer.

What he does is take a relaxation break. He leaves his office, walks outside, and watches the world around him. "For me," he says, "it has essentially the same effect as more formal methods."

Other people can get the relaxation effect—and the lower blood pressure—by listening to the sound of running water in a brook. Or watching the sunlight on the leaves of a tree. Or gazing at a fire in a grate.

Some people repeat Dr. Katcher's experiment, and get a tank full of fish. There are some twelve million fish tanks in the United States—"and there's a very good reason for that," says Dr. Katcher.

"It's a matter of finding what works for you," he prescribes. One way or another, there's a health bonus in taking a relaxation break for ten or fifteen minutes, twice a day. There are all sorts of ways to relax, formal and informal. Whether it's watching trees or a blue sky, trying the relaxation response, or even joining a class in transcendental meditation, they all have the same key element in common.

You are focusing outward, away from your private thoughts, away from other people, and toward some object of contemplation. As Dr. Katcher puts it, "You are having a dialogue with something pleasing in your environment."

Man's—and Woman's—Best Friend

There's a special and valuable dialogue that takes place with a dog, a cat, or some other pet. More and more doctors are encouraging certain patients to get a pet, and in some hospitals, animals are being brought in to "visit" with patients. The evidence is growing that a pet can be good for your mental health and thus for your blood pressure.

Talking with a pet is one form of speech that does not raise the blood pressure. Indeed, researchers are finding that touching and talking to a pet actually brings the pressure down.

About 85 percent of pet owners, according to surveys, do talk to their animals, and about 30 percent "confide" in them. About 80 percent say that they believe their animals understand what they're saying and feeling.

Talking to a dog or cat takes a different form than talking to another person. With most men and women, the speech is slower, more lilting when talking to a pet, and many people pause, as if waiting for the animal to answer or at least pay close attention.

Children have these same sorts of conversations with imaginary playmates. Some people "talk" to loved ones who have died. There is no chance of being judged or criticized or disagreed with in these one-way conversations, and that's part of the positive, relaxing effect.

Religious people have long known about this. It's part of the reward that some find in prayer. Now science is documenting that the reward is very real indeed.

Will It Work for You?

"Many people would rather take a pill," says Dr. Katcher. "In our society, they still believe that disease is something you cure with medicine or surgery."

The idea of treating mind along with body, especially for blood pressure, is a new one, but attitudes are changing. More and more people are concerned about a healthy diet. Growing numbers are out running, swimming, playing games, doing aerobics and other exercises. The popularity of today's ideas about diet and exercise is a cultural change. Especially as the evidence grows about how well it works, the same thing is beginning to happen about relaxation.

Yet if some patients are skeptical or impatient, so are many doctors. Some just don't believe in it; most are too busy to offer very much in the way of training in meditation. "If you want your doctor to work with you on this, you have to handle the dialogue carefully," advises Dr. Katcher.

If you have a diastolic of 120, any doctor, including Dr. Katcher, is going to want to prescribe what's quickest—a surefire drug. You could, though, talk to your physician about adding relaxation to that, to make the drug even more effective.

If your diastolic is hovering around 100, you may want to talk to your doctor about lowering it without drugs. You could say that you want to try relaxation, perhaps along with losing weight and doing some cardiovascular exercise. "You could tell the doctor you'd like to try it for a month," suggests Dr. Katcher. "If it doesn't work within that time, you'd agree to go on to something else that the doctor advises."

Most doctors would agree to that, thinks Dr. Katcher. And for most patients, a month is long enough to see some results with relaxation.

14. Don't Get Mad, Get Healthy

Suppose that . . .

- At the last minute, someone cancels an appointment with you, without giving a good reason.
- The job promotion you want goes to someone else.
- Your marriage partner forgets your anniversary.
- Your child knocks over a glass of milk.
- A friend has not returned your phone call.
- You find that vandals, perhaps teenagers, have knocked over your mailbox.
- Another car cuts in front of you in a line of traffic.
- The repairman arrives late, does a sloppy job, charges "too much."
- You're disturbed by the noise your neighbor is making.
- It's thirty minutes past your appointment time, but you're still waiting to see the doctor.

What makes you angry? How do you feel when it happens? What do you think to yourself? What, if anything, do you say—or perhaps shout—to the other person?

How you deal with anger may affect your blood pressure. There is no personality profile for high blood pressure, no special pattern of behavior that makes hypertensives different from other people. There is, though, new evidence of a link between angry feelings and a diastolic that's too high.

"Feeling a lot of anger and not expressing it can lead to high blood pressure." That's the new hypothesis, and there's growing support for it. Based on observation and clinical experience, some doctors and researchers now believe that you can manage your blood pressure better by learning to manage your anger better.

Dr. Raymond Novaco is working on this at the School of Social Ecology at the University of California at Irvine. Dr. Margaret Chesney, director of the Department of Behavioral Medicine at the Stanford Research Institute, has proposed a major study of this to the National Heart, Lung, and Blood Institute. Dr. David Burns, professor of psychiatry at the University of Pennsylvania School of Medicine and author of *Feeling Good: The New Mood Therapy,* is a pioneer in developing new ways to heal your emotions and improve your health.

How Anger Works

The emotion of anger, like other forms of stress, is expressed in physical ways. Your breathing speeds up. Your muscles tense. A frown forms on your face. And your blood pressure goes up.

If you often feel angry, that means your blood pressure will be going up often. If the anger stays with you, kept inside, kept alive, then the pressure will stay up, too.

Sometimes, anger feeds on itself. As the philosopher William James wrote, "One may get angrier in thinking over one's insult than at the moment of receiving it."

Anger has two directions to go, out or in. If you express it outwardly, at the person or thing that's making you angry, that's what's meant by releasing your anger. You're letting it go, though obviously some ways of doing that are better than others.

If you express it inwardly, you're directing it at yourself. You're holding on to it, brooding about it, letting it simmer. It's true what they say about anger. It does "burn you up." It does "eat you up inside."

People who keep their anger in are the ones who tend

to get in trouble with their blood pressure. If you're in this group, then Dr. Burns has a twofold prescription for you.

First, learn to reduce the amount of anger, the number of times you feel outraged or insulted.

And second, learn to express your anger outward, in appropriate ways.

A New Therapy

Why does one person see something as an insult, while another person takes it as a joke? Why does the same thing make you angry in one instance, when it passes by unnoticed in another?

Your anger depends on what you expect before the event, and how you interpret it afterward. That's the basis for Cognitive Therapy, a new psychological approach that doctors are using to help people deal better with emotions such as anger. Your cognitions are your inner thoughts, your private ways of knowing and seeing yourself and the world around you.

Sometimes, these inner thoughts can be irrational and even silly. Yet their effects can be very real and serious. Often, we're not fully aware of these inner thoughts. Yet if we can become more aware of them, we may be able to change some of them. We may be able to learn to see ourselves and other people in truer and healthier ways.

According to Dr. Burns, someone who suppresses angry feelings, holding them in, may be carrying on an inner dialogue that goes like this:

"I have no right to be angry."

"Anger is bad."

"If I show my anger, people will see that I'm a bad person."

"It's wrong to be angry at a husband . . . or a wife . . . or parent."

"Nice people in good relationships don't get angry with each other."

"If I express my anger, something bad will happen."

Do those thoughts seem foolish? If you're someone who doesn't express your anger, do they also seem familiar?

Think about those inner thoughts. Test them against reality. Maybe you can replace them with truer statements.

Maybe you can rewrite them, so that your inner dialogue now goes like this:

"Someone hurt me."

"I have a right to be angry."

"I have a right to my feelings, because I'm a worthwhile person."

"People who love each other don't always agree."

"If you argue with a husband . . . wife . . . or parent, it doesn't mean you don't love that person."

"If I attack or blame the other person, something bad could happen."

"If I share my feelings and my views about what's going on, something good could happen."

"Maybe we can work things out."

Your inner dialogue comes out of a lifetime of learning what's "good" and what's "bad." It takes practice to change it. In working with his patients, Dr. Burns has developed some exercises that can help.

Try this: Think of a recent time or two when you felt angry. Without worrying about whether they're foolish or not, write down as many thoughts as you can remember. Now test those thoughts against these questions:

Did someone hurt you? Knowingly? On purpose? Unnecessarily?

Is your anger directed against that person? Or against yourself?

Is your anger useful? If you expressed it, would it help you to reach a desired goal? Or would it hinder you?

On the basis of those answers, now try to rewrite your dialogue.

Why Are You Angry?

Along with the thoughts that keep you from expressing your anger, there are the thoughts that made you angry in the first place. Those, too, need looking at, to decrease the amount of anger you may feel.

Typically, when we feel angry, we feel that someone has gone against our values, our moral code, our personal rules, our inner guidelines. A friend forgets to call, and you think, "That's not how a friend is supposed to act." Or a stranger seems to be taking advantage of you. Or a boss fails to recognize your good work. Or a loved one wants something different than you do.

When those things happen, we think, "That's not fair!" Or, "That shouldn't have happened." Or, "That person has no right to do that or say that."

We want to defend our values, but we also need to learn to save our anger for those things we can do something about. Suppose, for example, that vandals have knocked over your mailbox. It's wrong; it's unfair. Can you find the vandals? Can you do something to prevent future vandalism? If so, then anger may have some use. If not, if you get angry and stay angry, you're letting the vandals hurt you twice—first in your mailbox and then in your emotions.

The anger-prone person tends to take things personally. So you may think, "They did that to *me*. They picked *me* out to hurt." Yet if you look down the street, are the other mailboxes bashed in, too? It's still wrong, but an impersonal insult is less infuriating.

What Are You Thinking?

It's not an event that makes us angry, but the way we interpret that event. Each of us has a private list of "should's" and "shouldn'ts" that we want other people to live up to. We have a sense of what we're entitled to, what we "deserve," and when we don't get it, we get angry. In an imperfect world, where what's fair isn't always what happens, we may need to rewrite some of those expectations and assumptions.

"Other people don't make you angry," explains Dr. Burns. "You make yourself angry, with your own thoughts." Suppose, for example, a wife is angry at her husband, because he wants to watch the football game on TV while she wants them to go out together. Her inner dialogue may be going something like this:

"If I'm a good and faithful wife, he should love me."

"If he loves me, he should always want what I want."

"He always wants his own way."

"If he prefers the football game, he doesn't love me."

"If he doesn't love me, it's because I'm not lovable or worthwhile."

"Or it's because he's a rat."

The dialogue may seem silly, but in the privacy of our minds, it's how many of us think. Notice the "hot" words like "should" and "always." Watch out for labeling and monster-making, calling people names like "rat." These are the ways we fan the flames of anger.

A more realistic dialogue would begin like this:

"If I'm a good and caring wife, he'll respond in a loving way a good bit of the time."

"When he doesn't, I can still feel worthwhile."

"Even if we love each other, we won't always want the same things."

"When we disagree, sometimes he gets his way and sometimes I get mine."

If the dialogue begins this way, it can end on a more positive note. The wife will feel better about her husband and about herself. She may find a way to express her feelings so that she gets what she wants—not always, but more often than before.

Your Anger Top Ten

Try another exercise from Dr. Burns. In his book *Feeling Good: The New Mood Therapy,* he suggests that you make a list of your "anger hierarchy," the ten things that make you the angriest. These can be personal events, big or small. They can include impersonal things, perhaps an outrage, such as a rape, that you read about in the newspaper.

Now write down the thoughts that you usually have about these things. Look at that inner dialogue. Can you improve on it? What thoughts could be changed? What is the goal you desire, and how can you get closer to it? Now write down your new inner dialogue.

The Do's and Don'ts of Anger

As you learn to think truer thoughts, there'll be fewer times when you feel anger. There will still be times, though, when the anger is there, sometimes rightly, sometimes wrongly, sometimes justified, sometimes not. When that happens, how do you express that anger?

If you hold it in, you're still expressing it, perhaps by overeating or overdrinking, probably in your blood pressure. If you direct it outward, how do you keep it from ricocheting?

If you lash out, battering the other person with words or blows, you're creating more anger and not doing much to solve the problem at hand. The trick is not to be aggressive but to be assertive.

The assertive arguer speaks up, but with reasonable calm. He or she stands up for his rights, but without trampling the other person; if you destroy your opponent, he'll want revenge one day.

For the assertive person, an argument is an occasion for sharing feelings, views, ideas, not for name-calling and mudslinging. Being assertive lets you get things off your chest, but it leaves room for the other person to present his or her side—and perhaps see yours.

Here, from cognitive therapists, are some guidelines.

Five Anger Don'ts

1. Don't take it personally.
2. Don't focus on the insult. Instead, concentrate on what you need to do to resolve the conflict or achieve your goal.
3. Don't exaggerate the importance of events. A single moment doesn't define an entire friendship, or marriage, or career.
4. Don't expect too much—of others or of yourself. Try to keep your assumptions and expectations reasonable.
5. Don't get caught by surprise. Learn to recognize the signs of anger in yourself. Do you clench your jaw? Can you feel tears building up? Are you breathing faster? Use those signs as cues to start coping.

Five Anger Do's

1. Do give yourself a moment. Take a breath, time enough to ask yourself, "Am I interpreting this event correctly? Or

is there another way of looking at it?" Take another breath, to monitor your inner thoughts.

2. Do use "I" statements. Instead of "You did such-and-such," try saying "I feel this-and-that."

3. Do be tactful, low-key, respecting of yourself and of the other person.

4. Do have a sense of humor. A joke can defuse your anger and the other person's. A funny mental image of the other person—perhaps in diapers—can ease the fear that may be part of your anger.

5. Do practice. If you're not used to asserting yourself, try it on a waiter or a salesperson before you try it on your boss. Or think of the situations you're likely to encounter, plan how to deal with them, and rehearse—on your own or with a friend.

Managing your anger isn't easy, and it won't happen overnight. Give it time. If you slip, be forgiving, not angry, with yourself.

15. Here's to Your Health!

In this book, we've been talking about the many different ways that you can control your blood pressure and lower it in thirty days.

Some of the cures are at the pharmacy.

Some are on the shelves of your supermarket.

Many are in your head.

They are there for the taking. In the end, it is up to each person to reach for them—singly or, better yet, in combination. The more of these ideas you try, the quicker your blood pressure will drop and the healthier you will be.

The tragedy of high blood pressure is that not everybody reaches out for help and health. People respond very differently to illness of any kind. Some feel fear, an emotion that makes almost any illness worse. Some try to pretend that nothing is happening. Some resign themselves to fate.

The wise ones feel curious. They take it as a challenge. They approach it with confidence. They enlist mind and body, each in the other's service. They use positive emotions to create a personal environment that makes any medical treatment work better.

As you follow any of the ideas in this book, something special is happening. You are coming to know and understand yourself. Like all knowledge, that's a kind of power. It may not seem to have much to do with blood pressure, yet it has everything to do with it.

Many of the ideas in this book are ways of taking control of your life. That's true whether it's dieting or exercising, stopping smoking or starting to use relaxation techniques, managing your sodium or managing your anger. As you do any one of those things, it adds to the sense of control and competence you need for any of the others.

There's a bonus, a plus, a great reward in that. That sense of control can spread and touch all the areas of your life. As you learn to control your blood pressure, you are adding years to your life—but you are doing more than that. You are adding fullness, goodness, new satisfactions to those years.

Start now. Decide that today will be the first day of that better life.

Index